Professional Skills in Nursing

Professional Skills in Nursing

A Guide for the Common Foundation Programme

Rita Debnath

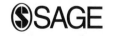

Los Angeles | London | New Delhi
Singapore | Washington DC

First published 2010

SAGE Publications Ltd
1 Oliver's Yard
55 City Road
London EC1Y 1SP

SAGE Publications Inc.
2455 Teller Road
Thousand Oaks, California 91320

SAGE Publications India Pvt Ltd
B 1/I 1 Mohan Cooperative Industrial Area
Mathura Road
New Delhi 110 044

SAGE Publications Asia-Pacific Pte Ltd
33 Pekin Street #02-01
Far East Square
Singapore 048763

Library of Congress Control Number: 2009926213

British Library Cataloguing in Publication data

A catalogue record for this book is available from the British Library.

ISBN 978-1-84787-396-5
ISBN 978-1-84787-397-2 (pbk)

Typeset by C&M Digitals (P) Ltd, Chennai, India
Printed and bound in Great Britain by TJ International Ltd, Padstow, Cornwall
Printed on paper from sustainable resources.

Mixed Sources
Product group from well-managed forests and other controlled sources
www.fsc.org Cert no. SGS-COC-2482
© 1996 Forest Stewardship Council
FSC

Contents

Acknowledgements   vi

Introduction   1

1   Study Skills   3

2   Health and Safety   11

3   Communication Skills   26

4   Infection Control and Standard Precautions   36

5   Hand Washing and Aseptic Technique   54

6   Vital Signs and Neurological Observations Monitoring   67

7   Hygiene Needs   88

8   Nutritional and Hydrational Needs   105

9   Elimination   123

10   Administration of Medicines   149

11   Administration of Injections   163

12   Wound Care   178

Answer Guide   195
Glossary   202
Bibliography   208
Index   216

Acknowledgements

I would like to take this opportunity to acknowledge and thank SAGE for their much needed input and for providing me with the direction required.

Every effort has been made to obtain the copyright holders but if any have been inadvertently omitted, the necessary arrangement will be made to amend the situation at the earliest opportunity.

Introduction

The Nursing and Midwifery Council (NMC 2008) states that 'nurses and midwives must provide a high standard of practice and care at all times' while also keeping 'knowledge and skills up to date throughout your working life'. Having a sound understanding of how the body functions and of medical conditions is essential but not sufficient as a basis for nursing. The pre-nursing curriculum includes such matters as ethics, research, technology, health education and health promotion. This is designed to help student nurses to be able to critically analyse their actions, thoughts, practice, clinical skills and apply these newly acquired processes, knowledge and clinical skills in practice. Student nurses will be equipped to improve their practice and demonstrate their understanding of the clinical skill being performed.

None of this occurs in a vacuum: nurses work not in isolation, but within a complex health and social care system. Numerous developments – for example, technological changes, the introduction of foundation status, changes in financial management, the introduction of the modern matron system – have affected the way nurses work.

This book focuses on the knowledge and skills that nurses need in order to respond and adapt to such changes effectively. Of central importance are the introduction of the *Essential Skills Clusters* (NMC 2007a) and *The Code – Standards of Conduct, Performance and Ethics for Nurses and Midwives* (NMC 2008: 7), which states that nurses 'must deliver care based on the best available evidence or best practice'. The Essential Skills Clusters are UK-wide generic skills statements, organised into five clusters – care, compassion and communication; organisational aspects of care; infection prevention and control; nutrition and fluid management; and medicines management. They apply to all branches of nursing and seek to address some of the concerns about skill deficits arising from the Review of Fitness for Practice (NMC 2007b). They are skills that support the existing NMC outcomes for entry to the branch programme, and the proficiencies required for entry registration (NMC 2007a). The Essential Skills Clusters (NMC 2007a) are not designed to encompass all the skills required to be proficient as a nurse. Instead, they concentrate on potential areas of deficit so the public can be assured that these are dealt with in every pre-registration nursing programme in the United Kingdom.

The book covers clinical skills within a pre-registration nursing programme, especially the common foundation programme of a three-year nursing programme. It both introduces the skills and seeks to provide a cognitive understanding of why each skill is performed. The book promotes an approach to nursing care that is holistic and evidence based. An holistic approach recognises every individual as a human being. Thus, this book encourages students to think about patient dignity, comfort, respect and the biopsychosocial needs of the patient in relation to the clinical skill.

Overall, the book aims to provide students with a firm foundation on which to build when progressing to their chosen branches of nursing. It aims to contribute to the development of nurses who 'must deliver care based on the best available evidence or best practice' (NMC, 2008: 7) 'so that new qualifiers are capable of safe and effective practice' (NMC 2007a: 1).

Each chapter deals with a number of key clinical skills identified within the NMC Essential Skills Cluster (NMC 2007a). No chapter has been given precedence over any other, though those on study skills and communication have been placed near the start of the book in order to encourage an holistic approach of the type outlined above. Each chapter applies the skills it discusses to patient care, with theoretical knowledge to explain the rationale behind each skill (that is, to explain the 'why' and not just the 'how'). Learning outcomes are listed at the beginning of each chapter to help the reader focus on what is to be learned. Chapter introductions contextualise the material to be covered, while end of chapter summaries recount the salient points. Each chapter is supplemented by activities to develop critical thinking skills, test the student's knowledge and understanding and help consider care being delivered. Each chapter is fully referenced. Explanations of terms given in the text are supported by a glossary at the back of the book.

References

NMC (2007a) *Guidance for the Introduction of the Essential Skills Cluster for Pre-Registration Nursing Programmes*. NMC, London.

NMC (2007b) *Review of Fitness for Practice*. NMC, London.

NMC (2008) *The Code: Standards of Conduct, Performance and Ethics for Nurses and Midwives*. NMC, London.

1

Study Skills

Learning Outcomes

This chapter is designed to help you:

- o   prepare yourself to study as effectively as possible
- o   identify ways of studying
- o   recognise different learning styles
- o   develop your skills in the areas of (a) note-taking (b) gathering information (c) writing essays and reports (d) giving presentations, and (e) doing exams
- o   understand the role of reflection in learning.

Introduction

Learning takes place in many different ways: it may happen either formally or informally – and students adopt various styles of learning. Learning can be fun and help students to solve problems, though it can also prove challenging, especially if the learner has not studied for a number of years. NMC (2007) specify that before entering the branch programme students should be able to demonstrate the literacy, numeracy and computer skills needed to record, enter, store, retrieve and organise data in the course of care delivery.

There are several study skills guides on the market designed to help students become more effective learners. These include Cottrell (2003), Peck and Coyle (2005a, 2005b). This chapter does not intend to replicate these guides by examining each approach to study in detail. Instead, it provides an overview designed to provide you with a starting point for developing yourself and your learning further.

There has been much research into students' learning and this has established a number of important points. Ladd (1999) and Angela and Riazantseva (1999), for example, argue that study skills support needs to be directly related to students' immediate and specific needs. Research shows too that developing readiness to learn, through preparation and planning, are important (Bastable 2003).

Readiness may be divided into four components: physical readiness, emotional readiness, experiential readiness and knowledge readiness. Bastable (2003) has identified a number of factors that affect learning. They include aim, fatigue, sensory deprivation, the ability to concentrate, motivation, attitude, past experiences of learning, cognitive ability and learning style. Identifying your preferences as a learner can help in developing an effective study plan.

Honey and Mumford (2007) have identified four types of learning style. Some people are activist learners. They thrive on, and develop from, new experiences. Typically they are open minded and enjoy problem-solving, group work, seminars and debates. They tend to learn less effectively from lectures, having to understand data, reading, watching, or listening. They dislike repetition and become bored easily. A second type are the reflectors. They prefer to work alone through observation and reflection, by standing back and listening. They prefer learning from lectures, individual study and project work, and enjoy producing reports and performing tasks. They learn less effectively from leading an activity, participating in role plays or working to deadlines. A third type consists of pragmatists. They like to learn from problem-solving, practical sessions and clinical experiences. They tend to be practically minded and impatient. They learn less effectively when there is no immediate or obvious benefit to them or when they are required to follow guidelines. Finally, there are theorists. They like to learn from structured situations with clear guidelines; they enjoy theoretical discussion and like to evaluate material. They tend to be perfectionists, detached, analytical and adaptable. They learn less effectively where situations are unstructured.

Identifying what kind of learning style works best for you will help you to learn more effectively. To do this, please see Learning Activity 1.1.

LEARNING ACTIVITY 1.1

There is a quiz on the 'Leonardo da Vinci' pages of the Science and Nature section of the BBC website. You can use the quiz, which is called 'What kind of learner are you?' to help to understand yourself as a learner. For the quiz, go to: www.bbc.co.uk/science/leonardo/thinker_quiz/

Studying can be daunting and there may be a number of obstacles to effective learning. These include: lack of a suitable environment (one that is not too noisy, is the right temperature and so on); demands on time and resources for study; negative images of learning and study; fear; lack of reward or immediate benefit from studying; lack of funds to be able to study; lack of motivation and confidence; lack of tutorial or personal support; lack of access to Higher Education Institutions (HEI) or Further Education (FE) or to courses in the right place at the right time.

Hull (1997a) has suggested that there are a number of strategies that learners can use to make good use of time and facilitate learning. They include:

- setting aside realistic time to study
- allowing time to relax
- allowing time for family and friends
- studying at times that suit you
- allowing more time for the areas you struggle with
- allowing time for research

- setting yourself deadlines to complete your work
- allowing for any last-minute unforeseen problems and if they occur, to stay focused
- working in groups to facilitate learning
- identifying the skills needed to facilitate learning
- identifying weaknesses that may hinder learning so strategies may be sought to overcome those weaknesses.

Several principles may be applied to your study. You can benefit from (a) reviewing work regularly (b) establishing a study and revision timetable to minimise unnecessary stress (c) making learning interesting by adopting a variety of different strategies. All of these can help you to become an effective lifelong learner.

There are a number of measures that institutions can take to promote effective study. Durkin and Main (2002) researched study skills support for first-year undergraduate students. They found that there was a 'definite demand for a discipline-based study skills course for undergraduates' (2002: 36) and that the course needed to be run in the first half of the year to enable a cyclical approach to the acquisition of study skills. They also found that students benefited from liaison between study skills tutors and lecturers concerning students' learning and from access to assignments and question papers, past and present.

Required Skills

Note Taking

Note taking in lectures has three purposes: it can help the student to recall lectures for the future, it can clarify material discussed during a lecture and it can aid concentration during lectures. Note taking can provide a useful record of important points for future use and of sources of information. Note taking can also help students with aspects of their writing (such as flow of ideas, planning and organising work), their understanding, their ability to summarise the salient points of a lecture, and with revision. It can be useful to develop a form of shorthand to help you take notes efficiently.

Information Gathering

The task of gathering information can be highly educational, not least because it requires students to make decisions over which pieces of information are relevant (Marland 1991). However, the task can be daunting. It is easy to waste time through inefficient searching and this can sap the learner's morale.

It is important to ensure that search engine terms are not too broad. For example, searching a database using just the term 'pain' is likely to be too general for any particular purpose and so leads to irrelevant sources. More precise searches (for example, using the terms 'pain' and 'childbirth' together) will produce more specific results. It is also important not to rely on a single information source – rather, seek to use a wide range. These may include library resources, books, journals, bibliographical databases (e.g., CINAHL), reports and sets of statistics.

Writing Essays

Many students find essay writing the most challenging aspect of higher education courses. The challenge is to produce essays that are accurate in content and well presented, well structured, well written and well referenced. It is important before writing to clarify what the essay question is asking and then to discard any information that is irrelevant.

Hull (1997b) has identified five main stages to essay writing. They are: choosing the essay topic (one that will challenge the student); defining the question (through, for example, highlighting key words, brainstorming ideas, rephrasing in your own words for greater clarity); doing your research and reviewing the sources (are they current, at the right level and of sufficient depth); organising material; and reviewing the content of the essay once written to ensure it has answered the question.

Cottrell (2003) has also produced a schema for essay writing. It consists of the following seven stages: clarify the question; plan and prepare the essay; research the content; reflect on and evaluate the content produced; proofread the draft and make the necessary amendments; produce the final essay and submit it; and consider all the feedback provided. If you have problems understanding the required content or direction of the essay *do not* feel ashamed in asking for help or guidance.

Presentations

If you are required to give a presentation, plan and structure it with a clear focus and ensure that you are clear over the length required (Hull 1997a). Consider the audience – both its likely size and composition. For example, if the audience is made up of fellow students you may well be presenting them with new information (so clarity will be especially important), whereas if it includes your tutors, they will already have a knowledge base in the subject (so you might include interactive material to keep them engaged).

When preparing a presentation, select and structure the content and decide the presentation methods to be used (e.g., video, role play). Structuring your material into an introduction, main body and a conclusion can help to produce a logical sequence for the audience to follow. Prompts and summaries to the audience about what you have covered, what you are discussing at each stage and what the presentation will go on to cover can help the audience to understand the material. Practise before delivering the actual presentation and aim to make your delivery enthusiastic and dynamic. Before the presentation starts, check that you have any presentation aids ready to hand and that they are in good working order. After you have given the presentation, remember to evaluate it.

Exams and Exam Preparation

The purpose of exams is to check your understanding of the work covered on the course. Examinations require focused, intensive learning. When preparing for an exam, ensure you know what it covers and what type of exam it is – for example, whether it is a 'seen' or 'unseen' paper. If the latter, clarify the format (for example, whether it consists of multiple-choice questions, short-answer questions or essay questions). Preparation is everything. Devise a timetable for regular revision to be done on your own or in groups. This will make study more structured and less stressful. Revise directly after taking notes of a lecture's salient points, after study sessions, after covering a topic, at the end of every term or before tutorial sessions in order to retain the information over a period of time. Relax (as stress decreases the ability to learn), replenish yourself (a balanced diet and hydration improve learning and results) and get plenty of sleep. Plan and practice in advance, using past papers where possible.

Honey and Mumford (2007) have identified a number of principles for exam preparation. They include: taking frequent short breaks (as the brain only remembers the first and last thing read); using acronyms or word associations to remember key points; reviewing notes and work continuously (as 70 per cent of what is learnt during one day's study is forgotten immediately the next day); allowing for plenty of sleep (as sleep allows the brain to recuperate); storing and filing information carefully (as this facilitates learning); and acknowledging mistakes you have made (as learning arises out of making mistakes).

On the day of the exam, eat well (eating slow-release carbohydrates releases energy slowly and consistently), ensure you know when and where the exam is, and give yourself plenty of time to get there. Once in the exam, take time to read the instructions and questions carefully and read them at least twice. Jot down a plan to ensure the question is answered fully and leave time to check your answers at the end of the exam (Cottrell 2003).

Writing Reports

Reports are written for a wide range of reasons (for instance, following an accident or critical event, presenting a research report). Table 1.1 outlines the various components of a report and their rationale.

Be disciplined about including only necessary information, be succinct and present findings that will engage, interest and stimulate the reader. Focus the report upon the reader's need, rather than your own (Hull 1997b).

Table 1.1   *Report writing*

Page	Rationale
Title page	Reflects the nature of the report and includes information such as names
Abstract	Used independently of the report as it contains key recommendations found in the report
Contents page	Contains the main themes of the study with page numbers, list of tables and appendices
Introduction	Sets out the study and includes how the study originated, why it was undertaken, significance of the issue being investigated and contributes to existing knowledge
Methodology	Describes the process used with justification to investigate the research
Findings	Presents the research issue easily, e.g., diagrammatically
Conclusion	Pulls the main parts together and summarises the study, discusses the value of the study in relation to change with a brief reference to any limitations
Recommendations	Includes the need for change or suggests areas for further study
Appendices	Included at the end if required
Bibliography	Distinguishes between 'nice to know' and 'essential' information

(Hull 1997b)

Experiential Learning

Studying and learning not only occur in university but also in clinical practice. Learning from experience while in clinical practice is an integral part of being a nurse. However, many students exposed to the clinical setting focus exclusively upon their academic achievement (for example, ensuring their documentation is completed for the university) rather than making the most of the opportunity to expand their knowledge base and learn experientially. Being exposed to a clinical setting raises a number of challenges: for example, balancing home life with the rigours of academic study, learning how to nurse in an alien environment (especially if there is no prior experience of nursing), coping with interpersonal dynamics within a multidisciplinary team, and having to implement skills taught in an academic setting within the realities of practice. One such approach that can facilitate the process is that of reflection. This is discussed below.

Reflection

Reflection is a process where an individual examines their experiences, values, behaviour and knowledge in order to produce a new understanding of a situation and their practice. It is a way of informing practice, creating learning and arriving at judgements about practice. Nurses are required to reflect upon practice as specified by the UKCC (1990, 1997), who expect all qualified nurses to be reflective and maintain portfolios. UKCC (1999: 38) later stated that pre-registration nurses must be able to 'demonstrate critical awareness and reflective practice'.

Conceptions of reflection vary. Dewey (1993) viewed reflection as thinking with a purpose, while Johns (2004) viewed it as a way in which a practitioner could look at themself and their own experiences, in order to resolve the difficulty experienced in practice.

A number of models of reflection have been proposed. Schon (1983) for example, saw theory and techniques as a way to solve problems in practice by 'reflecting in' and 'reflecting on' action, but failed to acknowledge the complex nature of clinical practice in which nurses worked. Boud et al. (1985) saw reflection as deliberate learning where experience is evaluated and a new perspective gained, while Gibbs (1988) related reflection to stages that help students develop reflective skills and new insights. As a model it helped develop self awareness, work through emotions and demonstrate evidence of learning through learning from experience. However, as a model it lacks analysis. Atkins and Murphy (1994) suggested that there were three key stages to reflection – an awareness of uncomfortable thoughts and feelings, critical analysis of uncomfortable thoughts and feelings, and creating a new perspective. However, Atkins and Murphy (1994) failed to take account of the positive thoughts and feelings which can also prompt reflection (Smith 1998). Taylor (2000) has suggested a number of tips to facilitate reflection: be spontaneous, express yourself freely, be open to ideas, choose a time of day that suits you, choose a reflective model that suits you, and find a critical friend who will challenge and provide feedback in a spontaneous manner. To develop this topic further refer to Learning Activity 1.2.

LEARNING ACTIVITY 1.2

Perform a web search for models of reflection. Consider the models found through your search. Select a model that you find easy to apply to your work.

No matter which reflective model is used, reflection provides a means of turning experience into learning in order to make the most of situations experienced and recognise their significance. The focus is on making sense of experience and drawing conclusions to improve practice. This can help students develop reflective thinking skills, order their thoughts (Rolfe et al. 2001), examine their own beliefs and challenge assumptions, ways of working and organisational structures. To develop this further, see Learning Activity 1.3.

LEARNING ACTIVITY 1.3

Using a reflective model that you feel comfortable with, reflect upon a recent incident which you were involved with in your practice area.

A) Evaluate what you would do differently, if anything, should you be involved in a similar incident again.
B) Consider what action could have been taken that may have been more helpful.
C) What specific things have you learnt and how will you apply that learning to your future practice?

Summary

In order to be successful in their study and learning students need to understand the process of learning, take responsibility for their own learning and full advantage of all the opportunities provided, in order to be a successful learner and to be aware of the factors that affect learning (e.g., motivation, readiness to learn) as well as the difficulties that can hinder learning (e.g., the environment, lack of time, child care, funds). Without these, effective studying and learning may not occur or result in a student being a lifelong learner.

References

Angela, M and Riazantseva, A (1999) If You Don't Tell Me, How Can I Know? *Written Communication* 16 (October): 495–525.

Atkins, S and Murphy, K (1994) Reflection: A Review of the Literature *Journal of Advanced Nursing* 18(8): 1188–1192.

Bastable, SB (2003) *Nurse as an Educator,* 2nd edn. Jones and Bartlett, Boston.

Boud D, Keogh R and Walker D (1985) *Reflection: Turning Experience into Learning.* Routledge Falmer, London.

Cottrell, S (2003) *The Study Skills Handbook,* 2nd edn. Palgrave, Basingstoke.

Dewey, J (1993) *How We Think: A Restatement of the Relation of Reflective Thinking to the Educative Process.* DC Health and Co, Lexington Massachusetts.

Durkin, K and Main, A (2002) Discipline-Based Study Skills Support for First Year Undergraduate Students, *Active Learning in Higher Education.* The Institute for Learning and Teaching in Higher Education and SAGE Publications 3(1): 24–39.

Gibbs, G (1988) *Learning by Doing: A Guide to Teaching and Learning Methods.* Further Education Unit, Oxford Polytechnic, Oxford.

Honey, P and Mumford, A (2007) *Campaign for Learning: What Kind of Learner Are You?* www.campaign-for-learning.org.uk/aboutyourlearning.htm

Hull, C (1997a) Developing Your Study Skills, *Nursing Times Learning Curve* 1(1): 14–15.

Hull, C (1997b) Improving Your Writing Skills, *Nursing Times Learning Curve* 1(2): 14–15.

Johns, C (2004) *Becoming a Reflective Practitioner.* Blackwell Oxford.

Ladd, P (1999) Learning Style and Adjustment Issues of International Students, *Journal of Education for Business* 74: 363–371.

Marland, M (1991) Skills for Independence, *Education Guardian,* 20 October.

NMC (2007) *Guidance for the Introduction of the Essential Skills Clusters for Pre-Registration Nursing Programmes.* NMC, London.

Peck, J and Coyle, M (2005a) *The Student's Guide to Writing: Grammar, Punctuation and Spelling,* 2nd edn. Palgrave Macmillan, New York.

Peck, J and Coyle, M (2005b) *Write it Right: A Handbook for Students.* Palgrave Macmillan, New York.

Rolfe G, Freshwater D and Jasper M (2001) *Critical Reflection for Nursing and the Helping Professions: A User Guide.* Palgrave, Hampshire.

Schon, DA (1983) *The Reflective Practitioner: How Professionals Think in Action.* Basic Books, New York.

Smith, A (1998) Learning About Reflection, *Journal of Advanced Nursing* 28(4): 891–898

Taylor, B (2000) *Reflective Practice: A Guide for Nurses and Midwives.* Buckingham, Open University Press.

UKCC (1990) *The Report of the PREP Project.* UKCC, London.

UKCC (1997) *PREP and You.* UKCC, London.

UKCC (1999) *Fitness for Practice: The UKCC Commission for Nursing and Midwifery Education* (Chair Sir Leonard Peach). UKCC, London.

2

Health and Safety

Learning Outcomes

This chapter is designed to help you:

o understand the importance of risk assessment and risk management
o gain an awareness of the legislation(s) currently in place to maintain safety in practice
o learn the basic principles of safe handling
o learn the basic principles of first aid and, in particular, of dealing with (a) burns and scalds, (b) poisons, (c) choking
o develop an awareness of the incidence of violence and aggression and how to deal with it
o be aware of professional responsibilities.

Introduction

Nurses have a **duty of care** to patients in their care. They are responsible for promoting and maintaining the health and safety of their patients as well as their own. This responsibility is wide-ranging: it includes, for example, assessing a patient's ability to eat and drink, maintaining a safe environment, assessing potential **risks** (such as broken equipment or trailing wires), administering medicines correctly, controlling infection, and minimising **hazards**. The effects of inadequate attention to risk are varied and potentially severe (Swage 2000). This chapter focuses on health and safety issues that arise as part of everyday nursing practice. The chapter also provides an outline of the principles of first aid. It covers emergency situations that are experienced in many different health care settings, such as burns and scalds, poisons, choking, and violence and aggression.

Risk Assessment and Management

The Health and Safety Executive (2003) has defined a risk as 'the chance, high or low that somebody will be harmed by a hazard'. NPSA (2007) considers risk as the probability that a specific adverse event will occur in a specific time period or as a result of a specific situation. According to the NMC (2008: 6), in order to manage risk you must act without delay if you believe that you, a colleague or anyone else may be putting someone at risk. You must inform someone in authority if you experience problems that prevent you working within this Code or other nationally agreed standards. You must report your concerns in writing if problems in the environment of care are putting people at risk.

Effective **risk management** must include a consideration of hazard. The Health and Safety Executive (2003) defined a hazard as 'anything that can cause harm', while NPSA (2007) viewed a hazard as a situation with the potential to cause harm. Nursing may involve dealing with several types of hazard, including: biological (e.g., bacteria, viruses, fungi, parasites); chemical; physical (e.g., sharps, dressings, linen, x-rays, machinery); psychological; and sociological hazards (e.g., those relating to mental health, social activities, or social class issues).

Nurses need to be able to identify potential causes of harm and to prevent harm from occurring. They need to act in accordance with NMC (2004) and the Health and Safety at Work Act (1974), which provides the legal framework designed to ensure high standards of health and safety in places at work. Central to the prevention of harm is the process of **risk assessment**. This needs to identify known or suspected risks, and any preventative measures already in place. It may then be used to produce an action plan, which will include precautions for the patient (HSE 2003).

During this process, four basic questions need to be considered:

- What can go wrong?
- How badly can it go wrong?
- How often might it occur?
- Is there a need for action?

A risk assessment can reduce the potential for harm and, in the process, improve the quality of work and care delivered, while also fostering innovation. This will help to ensure that practice complies with Standards for Better Health for England and Healthcare Standards for Wales (DH 2004a). Additionally, you must comply with the risk assessment procedures of your own trust.

The process of risk assessment should underpin every aspect of nursing care. It should be a systematic, deliberate and interactive process (Heaven and Maguire 1996). Assessments form an integral part of patient care and should be viewed as a continuous process (Cancer Action Team 2007). A thorough risk assessment can help to set priorities and improve decision making, and achieve an optimal balance of risk, benefit and cost.

The UKCC (1998) suggested risk assessment should cover patient care, the care system, and the local environment. The NMC (2004) states that nurses must 'act to identify and minimise risk to patients and clients'. To help understand risk assessment, refer to Learning Activity 2.1.

LEARNING ACTIVITY 2.1

While in placement:

- Make an assessment of potential hazards
- Make an assessment of potential accidents and who could be hurt by them
- Identify which hazards are indicated by signs
- Identify what procedures are in place to reduce hazard. Discuss your findings with your mentor.

LEARNING ACTIVITY 2.2

Within your placement area familiarise yourself with the policy pertaining to risk assessments. This may relate to specific risks or hazards such as:

- Falls
- Moving and handling
- Nutritional intake
- Pressure ulcer development
- Suicide risk assessment
- Maintaining a safe environment.

The Health and Safety Executive (2003) identifies risk assessment as an examination of factors that could cause harm to people in a care environment, conducted so that precautions can be taken to prevent injuries. This has five stages – looking for the hazard, deciding who may be harmed and how, evaluating the risks and deciding what should be done, recording the findings, reviewing the assessment and reviewing the outcome if necessary (NPSA 2007). It is impossible to eliminate risks and hazards completely but, by identifying risks, hazards and associated factors, the chances of harm occurring can be minimised.

Risk management is the process of identifying, assessing, analysing and managing all potential risks by adopting systematic assessment and review and seeking ways to prevent risk occurrence (NHSE 1999). NPSA (2007) defined risk management as assessing, analysing and managing risks, recognising which events (hazards) may lead to harm in the future, and minimising their likelihood and consequence. This applies to all aspects of nursing, including primary care, where risk is inherent in providing treatment and care, determining service priorities, giving instructions and dealing with patients (NPSA 2005).

According to NPSA (2005) clinical risk management is designed to:

- ensure the same system for managing risk is adapted regardless of the environment the health-care professional is working within
- ensure a consistent approach to risk assessments and improve information regarding risks
- help lessons learned in one area of risk to be applied to other areas
- provide a recognisable, safe, high quality service to patients, carers and public, and improve the quality of patient care
- reduce injury to patients and staff
- increase security and safety of equipment, buildings and people
- improve the healthcare environment
- reduce negligence claims.

Legislation

There are a number of health and safety laws in place to promote and protect health care professionals, the public and minimise hazards occurring. These include the Health and Safety at

Work Act (1974), which places specific responsibility upon employers to protect the welfare of people at work and the public, and Health and Safety at Work Regulations (HSE 1999). The provisions of the latter cover such issues as risk assessment, prevention of violence, accident monitoring, health surveillance, consultation with staff, effective management of risks, and provision of training. Other regulations include: Reporting of Incidents, Diseases and Dangerous Occurrences Regulations (RIDDOR) (HSE 1995); Provision and Use of Work Equipment Regulations (PUWER 1998); Lifting Operations and Lifting Equipment Regulations (LOLER 1998); and Moving and Handling Operation Regulations (HSE 1992, amended in 2002).

PUWER (1998) and LOLER (1998) were both designed to ensure that equipment used is suitable for use, well maintained, regularly inspected, only used by trained individuals and fitted with essential safety devices and warning labels (HSE 2002). They require electric hoists to be tested every six months and have the safe working load clearly marked on them. RIDDOR (HSE 1995) ensures accidents and **near misses** are documented and reported to the Health and Safety Executive (2002) so the accident can be investigated if necessary, and harm reduction measures implemented.

Safe Moving and Handling

Moving and Handling Operations Regulations (HSE 1992, amended in 2002) clearly lays out the responsibilities of employers and employees regarding moving and handling procedures and equipment use. The regulations highlight the need for training on a regular basis. Safe moving and handling requires avoidance of unnecessary handling, assessment of risk, and planning and preparing manoeuvres using the TILE (task, individual, load, environment) framework. This involves identifying and assessing the task (what is the job at hand – for example, moving a patient or inanimate object); individual (what can the health professional do for themselves); load (what can the patient do for themselves); and environment (is there enough room to undertake the task in hand).

When patients cannot move independently, moving and handling procedures must minimise the effort required for the handler and any discomfort experienced by the patient. Note in particular that back injury to the nurse is a common and sometimes serious occurence. BackCare (2001) estimated that £50 billion is lost per year to the United Kingdom economy due to back injuries, while DH (2004) stated that more than 11 million working days were lost each year due to back pain, costing £5 billion.

On completion of a risk assessment, the question of the most appropriate equipment to use may be considered. This must be consistent with the following guidelines – Health and Safety at Work Act (1974), Manual Handling Operations Regulations (HSE 1992), NMC (2002) and RCN (1993, 1996, 1999). A multidisciplinary team approach may be required to guide and encourage patients to assist the handler when being moved, as well as with their capabilitities for moving themselves.

Assessments of manual handling should be documented, acted on, reviewed and updated, with trained nurses attending mandatory updates. To help you become aware of the moving and handling assessment process, please refer to Learning Activity 2.3.

REFER TO PROCEDURE: MOVING AND HANDLING

LEARNING ACTIVITY 2.3

Locate your clinical area's Moving and Handling assessment form used for admission and ascertain how the form should be completed.

First Aid

First aid and emergency skills are part of the pre-registration programme. First aid refers to initial assistance or treatment provided before the arrival of qualified healthcare professionals. It often involves taking simple measures to save a life, prevent a condition from worsening, prevent further injury or promote recovery (Mohun et al. 2002). It may be administered by a member of the family, a friend, or stranger. What form is appropriate must be judged in relation to the circumstances and the knowledge and abilities of the person providing aid (NMC 2004). A core principle of first aid is that it should itself do no harm.

Table 2.1   *Action to be taken when first aid is required*

Action	Rationale
Assess the situation visually to ascertain what has happened, look for any dangers or potential hazards to yourself or patient	Important **not** to put self in any harm or danger so becoming the casualty
Once assessed clearly introduce yourself to the patient and ask what happened	Ascertains what happened
If unresponsive and environment safe assess airway, breathing and circulation/commence CPR and call for help – 999 or 2222 (within hospital)	Ensures professional help is contacted and arrives
Stay with the patient until professional help arrives and takes over	Prevents deterioration of patient condition

(Brooker and Waugh 2007)

Burns and Scalds

Burns can affect the two main areas of the skin, namely the **epidermis** and **dermis**. In severe cases the subcutaneous fat and muscle may also be affected. The main sources of burns and scalds are flames, steam, hot liquid or fat (DTI 2003), industrial and domestic chemicals, electricity and radiation. Burns may be classified according to depth and percentage of body surface area affected. The depth of burn injuries may be classified as superficial (the epidermis only is involved), partial thickness (the epidermis and dermis separate resulting in fluid filled blisters), or full thickness (dermal, subcutaneous layer and muscle are affected).

The extent to which burns affect the body is estimated by using the rule of nines for body areas. It divides the body into sections that represent nine per cent of the total body surface area. It can be used in conjunction with adult burn patients to determine the total body surface area that has been burned. The greater the area affected the greater the risk of shock caused by fluid loss. Medical attention should always be sought for burns affecting the face, groin, hands and feet. When more than 15 per cent burns in adults is present, hospital care is necessary. In children the figure is 10 per cent burns where a modified chart is used to calculate the extent of burns because of the different sizes of children (Fowler 2003).

LEARNING ACTIVITY 2.4

- Within your clinical area, find out about the rule of nines.
- Discuss with your mentor how it is used, if used at all.

For immediate treatment it is important to establish and maintain the patient's airway, breathing and circulation, cool the affected area under cold water, and remove jewellery and watches. Clothing stuck to the body should not be removed. The patient should then be transferred to hospital. Gels, sprays and butter are not recommended for cooling the burn. For large burns, the patient must be kept warm and non-adhesive dressings should be used for superficial burns, while partial/thick burns should ideally be covered with cling film. In the case of electrical burns, it is important to ensure that the power supply is switched off before the patient is attended to. The degree of burns should be assessed and urgent medical assistance sought as the electrical conductivity of the heart may be affected. For chemical burns, flush the burn with water, ensuring water flows away from the body in order to prevent further burns occurring. First aiders should remove the patient's clothing but should wear protective clothing themselves (such as heavy duty gloves and apron). It is important to ensure that paramedics are aware that chemicals were involved.

Patients who have sustained a burn caused by frostbite should be warmed from the inside using warm fluids slowly. The affected area should be warmed by using body heat, bathing in warm water and analgesia administered for pain relief.

Poisons

A poison is any substance entering the body in enough quantity to cause temporary or permanent damage. A poison may be ingested, inhaled, splashed or injected. Signs and symptoms will vary according to the poison involved, the amount taken and the route of entry. The general principle when treating poisons involves: establishing and maintaining the patient's airway, breathing and circulation; identifying the poison taken (is there a history of taking poison? Is there evidence of empty containers?) and identifying whether there is any drowsiness or loss of consciousness, nausea and vomiting. If a patient is unconscious, other injuries (such as bleeding) should be treated, professional help should be summoned, and the patient transferred to hospital.

Children naturally explore their environment with their hands and mouths. They are likely to seek out and swallow medicines (oral or otherwise) which they see adults taking, and may swallow non pharmaceutical products (e.g., cleaning fluids) if left easily accessible (Soloway 2000). No amount of warning or reasoning is likely to stop a child picking something up within easy reach. Therefore, substances such as drugs and cleaning fluids need to be locked up, out of the sight and reach of children, and child-resistant packaging should be used (Rodgers 1996).

If poisons have been ingested, protect the airway in case of vomiting. Do not induce vomiting. Use a pocket mask for resuscitation (if required) and refer to the Poison Centre. For inhaled poisons, breathing equipment will be required as the contaminant (carbon monoxide, gas, smoke) may still be in the atmosphere, so the emergency services should be called. The emergency services may contact the National Poisons Information Service (which has a 24-hour emergency helpline) and refer to the toxicology database of known poisons and recommended treatment.

Choking

Choking occurs when there is a partial blockage to the upper airway due to a morsel of food or foreign object becoming lodged in the upper airway. The signs of choking include struggling for breath, difficulty with talking, clutching or pointing to the throat, and cyanosed lips and mouth. Encouraging the patient to cough may be sufficient to dislodge and clear the obstruction. If this is not possible, it may be possible to dislodge the obstruction by providing five back slaps – checking between each back slap that the obstruction has been removed. If the patient is still choking, then five abdominal thrusts should be performed; after that, the whole process of back slaps and abdominal thrusts should be repeated.

If the patient becomes unconscious, perform abdominal thrusts by placing the individual on his or her back. Professional help should be sought (dialling 999 if in the community or 2222 in the hospital setting). If the patient is unconscious and not breathing, cardiopulmonary resuscitation (CPR) should be instigated and emergency help sought. Once breathing, the patient should be placed in the recovery position while awaiting the arrival of the emergency services.

Violence and Aggression

Aggression may take the form of an action or behaviour and may be physical (e.g., kicking, punching), verbal (e.g., insults, threats, allegations) or non-verbal (e.g., gestures). Non-physical violence includes verbal abuse (including racial or sexual insults), swearing, shouting, name-calling and bullying, insults, innuendo, deliberate silence, threatening gestures and postures, harassment, abusive phone calls and texts. RCN (2003) has viewed **violence** and **aggression** as a situation where a health professional experiences abuse, threat, fear or the application of force arising out of the course of their work.

Violent and aggressive incidents often arise when patients feel vulnerable. They may feel that violence or aggression is the only way to release their sense of stress or anger. A number of factors may precipitate violence or make its incidence more probable. They include: a history of violence on the part of the patient; illness (including mental health problems); head injuries; **hypoxia**; endocrine disorder causing confusion; anxiety; tiredness; pain; the use of drugs and alcohol; mental distress (e.g., paranoia); lack of information; lack of structured activity; noise, and heat. These factors are pertinent to all sections of healthcare. Austin (2001) lists healthcare professionals working in the community, mental health settings, the ambulance service, General Practice, acute settings, or emergency departments as those at highest risk of suffering violence. Leather (2002) also stated that all healthcare professionals were at risk of some form of aggression. Statistics from RCN (2005) show that 77 per cent of emergency department nurses reported being victims of violence and aggression during 2005–2006. The figures for ward and care home nurses were 52 per cent and 48 per cent respectively.

Violence is a subjective phenomenon: it may be interpreted in different ways. Garnham (2001) viewed violence as a serious physical attack with the intention of causing harm: it may be directed against either objects or people. Wright et al. (2002) viewed violence as 'acts in which there is use of force to attempt to inflict personal harm'.

It is important to identify the cause of the violent incident to understand why it has occurred and to differentiate between a conscious malicious incident and an unintentional violent incident.

A zero tolerance approach to violence and aggression will help to support nurses so that they can deliver care for patients safely. Garnham (2001) believed a systematic approach could empower the nursing workforce to regain the environment and develop the skills and understanding required to deal with the problem of violence. This approach is supported by documents such as Health and Safety at Work Act (1974) and Employment Rights Act (Department of Employment 1996).

Professional Responsibilities

Violent and aggressive situations can have a detrimental effect upon healthcare professionals. Some clinical areas are more susceptible to violent or aggressive behaviour than others. For instance, those working in Emergency Departments are susceptible to physical harm from those with mental health problems or those under the influence of alcohol or drugs, while those working on the ward are susceptible to verbal aggression from visitors or relatives. Dalphond et al. (2000), O'Connell et al. (2000) and Hesketh et al. (2003) identified that nurses were more likely to experience aggression from patients to whom they had given direct care and from visitors, relatives or friends, than were the multidisciplinary team (Rippon 2000).

Healthcare professionals have seen a huge rise in incidents of violence or aggression. According to the National Audit Office (2003), NHS staff in the UK reported 116,000 violent or aggressive incidents during 2000–2001. Studies suggest that acts of violence against NHS staff are still being unreported (Arnetz and Arnetz 2000, Rippon 2000, Beech 2001, Paterson et al. 2001).

Risk assessment will help to identify how and why violence might occur and consider what measures need to be taken to reduce the risk of such an event occurring. NICE (2005) states that the assessment involves identifying and controlling the environment, organisation, situation and staff attitude. This means ensuring the environment remains safe, ensuring structured and sensitive interviews occur to ascertain the trigger of the violent incident, ensuring the multidisciplinary team are involved in any risk assessment undertaken and demonstrating cultural awareness so as not to misinterpret any behaviour as being aggressive or violent.

Nurses therefore need to be aware of the factors that contribute to a violent or aggressive situation and to use their interpersonal and communication skills to try and defuse such situations. This may be referred to as 'conflict resolution' and Brandt (2001) suggested ways to assist this process – listening actively, not interrupting or being defensive, repeating comments objectively, requesting suggestions for dealing with the problem, examining options and deciding upon the best approach and, finally, adopting an open and honest discussion of any misunderstandings.

Employees can help to prevent incidences of violence and aggression from escalating by being empathic when communicating with the patient. This helps to calm them down. Colleagues need to ensure they are aware of and understand the situation, using observational and interpersonal skills (e.g., maintaining eye contact and adopting a calm, non-threatening approach) to diffuse the situation. By doing so the patient is being respected and not being denigrated or patronised. Withdrawing from the situation and moving people away from the situation to minimise harm to self and others, discussing the situation on a one-to-one basis in a calm, reassuring manner helps convey concern and can help resolve the situation.

To ensure safety, inform colleagues of your whereabouts and ask for help when necessary. In the community, mobile phones may be used to maintain contact with colleagues to ensure they are aware of your location. It also helps to travel in pairs. Informing emergency services, the GP or social services if visiting patients or areas known to present a risk to personal safety is essential for the aforementioned reasons.

REFER TO PROCEDURES: PREVENTION AND MANAGEMENT OF VIOLENCE (AND AGGRESSION)

NHS providers are obliged to protect their employees and develop strategies to reduce the number of violent and aggressive incidents towards nurses and healthcare professionals, as employers have a duty of care to identify and take preventable measures (Health and Safety at Work Act 1974, Dobson 1999). This can be achieved through employers undertaking a risk assessment to ensure the environment is one in which care can be delivered. An awareness of local trust violence and aggression policy is therefore required on the part of employees and students alike.

To reduce the risk of a violent and aggressive incident occurring employers can:

- install CCTV, glass screens, key-coded or swipe card doors, and panic buttons
- ensure that natural lighting is available and that everyone is aware that hospitals operate a smoke-free environment and that smoking is not allowed
- ensure that secure areas are available for mental health patients and victims of domestic violence
- create a calm environment
- implement policies and procedures to identify potential violent attacks
- provide training on de-escalation and break-away techniques for staff.

Should a violent or aggressive incident occur, it is important to record the incident, provide first aid and provide a debriefing session(s) for the team (and long term counselling and psychological support if required). Reporting to the police should be offered where a violent incident has occurred, as well as drawing up an agreement with the patient and healthcare professional. Having 'time out' or seclusion for short periods may be effective in mental health nursing. Locking doors, withholding treatment, restraining or forcing treatment are ethically and legally controversial in view of the Human Rights Act.

Seeking to adopt a calm, self controlled and confident manner while showing respect, empathy and professionalism is difficult, but in doing so it may be possible to prevent a delicate situation from turning into one that is out of control. Clear communication and confidence are essential here. It is always important to ensure that there is a debriefing session to discuss how a situation was handled. This should include a consideration of how basic interpersonal skills, such as tone of voice, attitude, posture and body language were used since, if used well, such skills can help diffuse violent and aggressive situations.

Summary

This chapter discussed the need for, and professional obligation towards, health and safety within practice. Acquiring and developing core safety skills is essential. Attempts should continually be made to reduce harm in healthcare, beginning with a generic (relating to patients, staff or a task) and specific (individual needs) risk assessment, as well as monitoring and adhering to legal obligations. Having a knowledge base of skills, such as moving and handling and first aid requires a questioning approach to be developed using evidence-based practice, reflection and an awareness of health and safety legislation which governs practice.

PROCEDURE: MOVING AND HANDLING

Action	Rationale
Assess: the patient's abilities/needs; task to be undertaken; your abilities; environment	To ascertain task to be undertaken; what your patient can do for themselves; what you are able to do; what the environment is like and what equipment is required for the task in hand
Document and inform the results of the assessment	To ensure everyone understands the results of the assessment; plan of care and coordinate task effectively Promotes and maintains privacy and dignity
Prepare the environment for the task, e.g., move lockers, chairs, draw curtains	To provide an ergonomic environment to manoeuvre and perform the task
Select the appropriate equipment in accordance with your assessment and training programme	To ensure safe moving and handling with little effort and minimal discomfort to the patient
Prepare and assist the patient into position with equipment for the task by using clear instructions and communicating with everyone Adopt a stable stance with knees bent slightly, keeping load close to the handler's body (where possible) and body in alignment	To prevent strain to all handlers and equipment takes all the strain Ensure everyone involved knows what to expect and therefore cooperates with the task Avoids stretching, straining, twisting, bending and keeps the back in natural alignment
Ensure patient comfort after performing the task; return those items removed; place call bell/patient items close to hand; store the equipment away and document all information	To evaluate task and method used and maintain a safe environment

PROCEDURE: ASSESSMENT OF VIOLENCE (AND AGGRESSION)

Action	Rationale
Multidisciplinary assessment of patient risk of becoming violent, e.g., neurological disorders or impairment; alcohol or substance abuse; previous history of violence or aggressive behaviour; stress; endocrine disorders	To reduce risk of a violent situation and avoid violence arising
Assess situations which may precipitate aggressive behaviour, e.g., washing, feeding	Ascertain if aggression precipitated by nursing care and therefore take appropriate action to reduce the risk of aggressive behaviour
Observe for any potential signs of aggressive behaviour, e.g., increased agitation; aggressive language; thigh tapping; fist clenching	To ascertain if patient is at risk of becoming violent

PROCEDURE: PREVENTION OF VIOLENCE (AND AGGRESSION)

Action	Rationale
Minimise the risk of violence and promote a safe environment by - ensuring staff are aware of the potential violent situation - not encroaching upon the individual's personal space or cornering them - keeping other patients out of the area - identifying a clear exit from the situation - observing for any potential weapons - appearing calm, relaxed, confident; and not appearing confrontational	To maintain a safe environment and avoid aggravating the situation
Talk clearly and quietly. Don't argue or become defensive Do not stare but be attentive Address the patients by their name and introduce yourself by your name	Arguing or being defensive may precipitate a violent situation. A calm approach may calm the situation; allow the patient the opportunity to express their anger which will enable you to ascertain the reason for their anger Staring can be interpreted as being domineering Being attentive and introducing yourself can help orientate the patient and demonstrates respect
Ask open questions, i.e., how, when	Helps to clarify the problem. Asking 'why' may provoke the situation
Problem solve to reduce the frustration and carry out actions with the patient's cooperation	Helps diminish anger in order to deal with the patient

PROCEDURE: MANAGEMENT OF VIOLENCE (AND AGGRESSION)

Action	Rationale
Be aware of long nails/hair; pens; badges which should be removed	Minimises the risk of physical injury to others, e.g., patients, staff
Call for assistance	Easier to manage the situation and alerts others to the situation
Lead others away from the situation	Violent incidents are distressing and may lead to violence

Action	Rationale
Senior nurse to assess the situation and ascertain if more trained staff in violence management techniques are required	To contain and manage the situation
When help arrives organise the situation by briefing them	Staff need to be informed to enable them to manage the situation
Call for medical help and prepare medication as required	Medication may be required to manage the patient, i.e., calm them down
If patient restraint is required give clear instructions and coordinate this Minimise discomfort	Staff must know the trust policy for restraint and provide a cohesive approach Restraint used for safety reasons not as a punitive measure
Restraint may be removed gradually as the patient calms down and is assessed as so	Patient may still be likely to strike out
Staff should withdraw from the patient gradually, leaving someone to stay with the patient	Gradual withdrawal is safer in case of further outbursts To observe the patient's mood, behaviour and provide reassurance

FOLLOW UP	
Action	**Rationale**
Attend to any injured patients/staff informing them of their leagal rights	Provide care and complies with legal obligations and hospital policy
Document the violent/aggressive incident	Complies with legal obligations and hospital policy
Debrief staff	Evaluate care, vent feelings and reflect upon the situation

References

Arnetz, JE and Arnetz, BB (2000) Implementation and Evaluation of a Practical Intervention Programme for Dealing with Violence Towards Healthcare Workers, *Journal of Advanced Nursing* 31(3): 668–680.

Austin, J (2001) Violence and Aggression: Managing the Risk to NHS Staff, *Health Service Manager Briefing*. No. 66 Croner Surrey.

BackCare (2001) UK Charter for Back Care www.backpain.org

Beech, B (2001) Sign of the Times of the Shape of Things to Come? A Three Day Unit of Instruction on 'Aggression and Violence in Health Settings for all Students During Pre-Registration Nursing Training', *Nurse Education Today* 9(8): 610–616.

Brandt, MA (2001) How to Make Conflict Work for You, *Nursing Management* 32(11): 32–35.

Brooker, C and Waugh, A (eds) (2007) *Foundations of Nursing Practice: Fundamentals of Holistic Care*. Mosby, Edinburgh.

Cancer Action Team (2007) *Holistic Common Assessment of Supportive and Palliative Care Needs for Adults with Cancer: Assessment Guidance,* Cancer Action Team, London. In Dougherty, L and Lister, S (2008) *Royal Marsden Hospital Manual of Clinical Nursing Procedures Student Edition,* 7th edn. Blackwell, Oxford.

Dalphond, D et al. (2000) Violence Against Emergency Nurses, *Journal of Emergency Nursing* 26(2): 105.

Department of Employment (1996) Employment Rights Act DH, London.

DH (1997) *The New NHS: Modern Dependable*. DH, London.

DH (2004) *Prevalence of Back Pain in Great Britain*. DH, London.

DH (2004a) *Standards for Better Health for England and Healthcare Standards for Wales*. DH, London www.dh.gov.uk

DTI (2003) *24th (Final) Annual Report of the Home and Leisure Accident Surveillance System 2000–2002 Data*. DTI, London.

Dobson, F (1999) *Dobson Steps up Major Drive to Protect NHS Staff from Assaults Violence and Security Memo from NHS Executive*. Stationary Office, London.

Dougherty, L and Lister, S (2008) *Royal Marsden Hospital Manual of Clinical Nursing Procedures Student Edition,* 7th edn. Blackwell, Oxford.

Fowler, D (2003) The Assessment and Classification of Non-Complex Burn Injuries, *Nursing Times* 99(25): 46–47.

Garnham, P (2001) Understanding and Dealing with Anger, Aggression and Violence, *Nursing Standard* 16(6): 37–42.

Health and Safety Executive (1992) *Moving and Handling Regulations*. Stationary Office, London.

Health and Safety Executive (1995) *Reporting of Injuries, Diseases and Dangerous Occurrences Regulations (RIDDOR)* DH, London.

Health and Safety Executive (1999) *Management of Health and Safety at Work Regulations: Approved Code of Practice and Guidance*. Stationary Office, London.

Health and Safety Executive (2002) *Simple Guide to the Provision and Use of Work Equipment Regulations 1998*. HSE, Sudbury.

Health and Safety Executive (2003) *Five Steps to Risk Assessment*. HSE, Sudbury.

Health and Safety at Work Act (1974) HMSO, London.

Heaven, CM and Maguire, P (1996) Training Hospital Nurses to Elicit Patient Concerns, *Journal of Advanced Nursing* 23: 280–286. In Dougherty, L and Lister, S (2008) *Royal Marsden Hospital Manual of Clinical Nursing Procedures,* 7th edn. Blackwell, Oxford.

Hesketh, KL et al. (2003) Workplace Violence in Alberta and BC Hospitals, *Health Policy* 63(3): 311–321.

Leather, P (2002) *Workplace Violence: Scope and Global Context*. In Cooper, C and Swanson, N (eds) *Workplace Violence in the Health Sector*. International Labour Organisation, Geneva.

LOLER (1998) *Lifting Operations and Lifting Equipment Regulations 1998.* HSE, Sudbury.

Management of Health and Safety at Work Regulations (1999).

Mohun, J et al. (2002) *First Aid Manual,* 8th edn. Dorling Kindersley, London.

National Audit Office (2003) *A Safe Place to Work: Protecting NHS Hospital and Ambulance Staff from Violence and Aggression.* NAO, London.

NICE (2005) *Violence: The Short Term Management of Disturbed Violent Behaviour in Psychiatric In-Patient Settings and Emergency Department.* NICE, London.

NHSE (1999) *Clinical Governance in London Region, Draft Template of Audit Risk Management Report for a Trust Board.* NHSE London Region, London.

NMC (2002) *Code of Professional Conduct.* NMC, London.

NMC (2004) *Code of Professional Conduct.* NMC, London.

NMC (2008) *The Code: Standards, Performance and Ethics for Nurses and Midwives.* NMC, London.

NPSA (2005) *Step Three Seven Steps to Patient Safety for Primary Care. Integrate Your Risk Management Activity.* NPSA, London.

NPSA (2006) *Risk Assessment Overview.* NPSA, London.

NPSA (2007) *Healthcare Risk Assessment Made Easy.* NPSA, London.

O'Connell, B et al. (2000) Nurses' Perceptions of the Nature and Frequency of Aggression in General Ward Settings and High Dependency Areas, *Journal of Clinical Nursing* 9(4): 602–610.

Paterson, B et al. (2001) Zero in on Violence, *Nurse Management* 8(1): 16–22.

PUWER (1998) *The Provision and Use of Work Equipment Regulations.* HSE, Sudbury.

Rippon, TJ (2000) Aggression and Violence in Health Care Professions, *Journal of Advanced Nursing* 31(2): 452–460.

RCN (1993) *Code of Practice for Handling of Patients.* RCN, London.

RCN (1996) *Code of Practice for Handling of Patients.* RCN, London.

RCN (1999) *Code of Practice for Handling of Patients.* RCN, London.

RCN (2003) *Dealing with Violence Against Nursing Staff: An RCN Guide for Nurses and Managers.* RCN, London.

RCN (2005) *At Breaking Point? A Survey of the Well Being and Working Lives of Nurses in 2005.* RCN, London.

Rodgers, GB (1996) The Safety Effects of Child Resistant Packaging for Oral Prescribed Drugs: Two Decades of Experience, *JAMA* 275: 1661–1665.

Soloway, RAG (2000) Poison Prevention: Messages and Resources, *Journal of Pharmacy Practice* 13(1): 33–36.

Swage, T (2000) *Clinical Governance in Health Care Practice.* Butterworth Heineman, Oxford.

Taylor, D (2000) Student Preparation in Managing Violence and Aggression, *Nursing Standard* 14(30): 39–41.

UKCC (1998) *Guidance for Clinical Healthcare Workers. Protection Against Infection with Bloodbourne Viruses. Recommendations of the Expert Advisory Group on AIDS and Advisory Group on Hepatitis.* DH, Wetherby.

Wright, S et al. (2002) *The Recognition, Prevention and Therapeutic Management of Violence in Acute In-Patient Psychiatry: A Literature Review and Evidence Based Recommendations for Good Practice.* UKCC, London.

3

Communication Skills

Learning Outcomes

This chapter is designed to help you:

o   understand what is meant by communication
o   understand why communication needs to be effective to care for patients and maintain a
    professional image
o   understand the use of interpersonal communication skills
o   be aware of barriers to communication
o   appreciate the role of record keeping.

Introduction

Communication is a powerful, potentially life changing activity. The NHS Plan (DH 2000) recognises communication as an essential and important part of nursing care. Chant et al. (2001) found that effective communication in healthcare influences patient satisfaction, compliance, complaint rates and levels of psychological and emotional distress. Campbell (2006) identified poor communication as one of the commonest causes of complaints in healthcare. DH (1999), UKCC (1999, 2000), ENB (2000) have all recognised the potential benefit of effective communication. UKCC (2000) identified communication as a core component of the knowledge base for nursing, which is confirmed by the NMC (2007: 2) Essential Skills Clusters, which state that in order to progress to branch one of the outcomes students must be able to 'engage in, develop and disengage from therapeutic relationships through the use of appropriate communication and interpersonal skills'.

Language has many roles. It is used, for example, to comfort, to socialise, to establish roles and also to restrict or punish behaviour (e.g., reprimanding a naughty child). Sensitivity to the communication process is an important aspect of working with patients and colleagues.

Poor communication and interpersonal skills can result in giving offence to colleagues as well as patients, so potentially damaging professional relationships (with possible negative impacts on patient care). Shrubb (2001) has highlighted the need to improve communication and record keeping in order to both prevent complaints and avoid clinical negligence.

Communication

The biological basis of communication lies in the sensory organs, while the interpretation of language and non-verbal signals (such as gestures and facial expressions) occurs in the brain. During spoken communication the sender transmits a message from the brain via the organs involved in voice production (the larynx, tongue, palate and lips) to the receiver. The receiver picks up the message through their ears, which is then transmitted to the brain via the vestibulocochlear (auditory) nerves. The receiver can then react and respond to the message.

Effective communication requires an awareness of the impact of personal and social factors. Such factors include: age, illness, disability, gender, culture, class, society, ethnicity and the environment. Use of jargon, slang, an unfamiliar accent, anxiety, fear, stress, anger and mental health problems can hinder communication.

Such difficulties require a variety of strategies. For example, patients experiencing anxiety, fear or stress may first require reassurance. For patients for whom English is not the first language, particular care needs to be taken over the use of medical jargon. In addition, an interpreter may be required.

Various models have been proposed to explain how communication works. Lasswell's model considers what is being communicated; who is communicating; with whom; what the channel of communication is; and what the effect of communication is. Neurolinguistic programme (NLP) models include a focus on the various ways in which people understand the world around them and how this influences people's communication and responses. Language, the senses, experiences, beliefs and values all influence the ways in which people communicate and how they interpret information.

Interpersonal Communication Skills

Communication is a reciprocal process – one that involves the exchange of verbal and non-verbal messages conveying feelings, information, ideas and knowledge (Wilkinson 1999, Wallace 2001). It is important to remember that **non-verbal communication** is an important part of the communication process (it perhaps accounts for 60 per cent or so of communication). Non-verbal communication is delivered through a variety of forms of body language (for example, gestures, posture, and facial expressions). It is used for a variety of reasons – for example, to express how people feel, express intimacy, establish control or dominance, or regulate interaction (by, for example, stopping someone talking).

If sensory processes are impaired it can result in communication difficulties. Those who are visually impaired might wear glasses, use Braille, and use large print text to communicate. Those with significantly impaired hearing might use lip reading and finger spelling. When speaking to a hearing-impaired patient, reducing the noise in the environment, ensuring hearing aids work, speaking normally, keeping hands away from the face, avoiding complex words and repetition can help with communication (see www. rnid.org.uk).

Egan (2002) has provided the acronym SOLER to summarise the elements of non-verbal communication. SOLER refers to:

- facing the patient **s**quarely
- maintaining an **o**pen posture
- **l**eaning slightly towards the patient to convey interest
- having appropriate **e**ye contact (neither not staring nor avoiding the patient)
- being **r**elaxed.

These measures encourage patients to communicate more openly. They are particularly important when dealing with communication-impaired patients, for example those who have suffered a stroke. Allowing plenty of time to communicate and not rushing helps to minimise feelings of frustration and isolation and to maximise successful communication.

Healthcare professionals and nurses need to assess a patient's communication needs and be attuned to their cultural beliefs. Offence can occur with inappropriate eye contact or touching, so sensitivity is required here. NICE (2004) suggest that suitably trained interpreters and advocates are made available to help overcome such difficulties.

LEARNING ACTIVITY 3.1

A child from another country has been admitted to your ward. English is not the child's first language making communication difficult.
  Drawing on your studies and experience to date, how would you seek to overcome this problem?

LEARNING ACTIVITY 3.2

You are placed on a mental health ward where patients have varying degrees of dementia.
  Drawing upon your studies and experience to date how would you communicate with such patients?

Barriers to Communication

Although current NHS policy, as confirmed by the NHS Plan (DH 2000) and NMC (2007) regards communication as an essential and important part of nursing care, there is often inequity in the way communication occurs in practice. For example, be careful not to assume that people from different cultures speak certain languages or necessarily require an interpreter. Instead, ascertain what language the patient uses and how they prefer to communicate. This will help to prevent misunderstandings, misdiagnosis, mistreatment and as a result, health suffering. A variety of means of communication may be used. They include questioning, interviewing, assessing patients, teaching, health promotion, the provision of information and accurate record keeping. It is important too to be an active listener. This will help you understand how and why people communicate the way they do, to identify what language is used and to understand a person's non-verbal communication. Listening is just as important as talking in helping to assess patient problems, needs and resources (Ravazi and Delvaux 1997).

It is also important to assess the impact of treatment and care provided: some medication (for instance, cloxapine) can impair communication by, for example, drying the mouth or causing excess salivation. (This may also lead to embarrassment, thereby affecting the patient's willingness to communicate. Take care to remain non-judgemental.) In this example, encourage fluid intake and provide mouth care to promote and facilitate verbal communication.

A number of barriers may prevent effective communication. These include lack of skill and understanding, undervaluing the importance of communication, lack of confidence, human failings (such as anxiety, stress, tiredness) and the working environment (for example, an exclusive focus on 'getting the work done'), among others. Noise (whether internal and external) can also hinder effective communication, overloading the brain with stimuli so that it can no longer process information. It is important to choose the time as wisely as possible to communicate with the patient (for example, when they are not distressed, anxious or angry) and ensure the environment is as conducive to communicating as possible.

Difficulty in hearing or with speech following a stroke or head injury can also hinder communication. In these cases, use drawing, writing, picture cards and signing. Refer the patient to the audiologist or **Speech and Language Therapist** (SALT). For those patients whose first language is not English or whose language has not developed (children), use an interpreter or play therapist. To help understand this further, work through Learning Activity 3.3.

LEARNING ACTIVITY 3.3

You have a patient with a hearing difficulty and you are finding it difficult to complete a full assessment.

- What resources are available within your clinical environment to help you?
- Would you involve anyone from the multidisciplinary team to help you? If so, whom?

Wilkinson (1994), Maguire et al. (1996) and Heaven and Maguire (1997) have all shown that nurses are often not proficient in communicating with their patients or identifying their difficulties. The problem may arise from nurses focusing upon physical and task-related aspects of nursing, from nurses' limited education and/or from a lack of training in communication (Chant et al. 2002). There is also evidence that nurses do not always communicate well with colleagues and other health professionals (Audit Commission 1993, Booth et al. 1996, Farrell 1996, Ashmore 1999). Nurses need to listen actively, display empathy and use straightforward language when performing everyday physical tasks.

Consider the skills required in the situation outlined in Learning Activity 3.4.

LEARNING ACTIVITY 3.4

A psychiatrist has prescribed a course of ECT for your client. The client is fearful of having ECT because of the stigma associated with ECT. You have built a good professional working relationship with the client.
    From your studies and experience to date, how would you deal with this situation?

LEARNING ACTIVITY 3.5

Choose a handover, ward round or case conference. Observe:

- How communication occurs
- Who the dominant figure is.

Care needs to be taken to avoid communicating in a patronising way. For example, when dealing with children or older people it is important to avoid patronising the patients through pats on the head or using words such as 'lovey'. Instead, the communication process should recognise the patient's knowledge, what they want to know, who they want to talk to and how much information they want to be given at any particular time. Checking patients' views, preferences and needs is paramount in order to create the optimal environment. But remember too, when the patient is a child or older person, that such factors as a patient's family context, the child's developmental level, usual family communication patterns and their past experience(s) with illness and hospitals are also important (Goldenberg and Goldenberg 1996, Lansdown 1996, Edwards and Davis 1997).

Record Keeping

Documentation and record keeping are integral to all aspects of nursing and healthcare, professional practice, and personal professional development (NMC 2005). It should be noted that documents and records are used for legal and auditing purposes. Medical records should be kept in a similar way to police records: pages and lines should not be left blank; erasers and tippex should not be used, and any mistakes should have a line drawn through (Faugier et al. 1997). Records should be made clearly and logically: they should not be open to misinterpretation and should be free from error. Should errors occur, they should be indicated appropriately (NMC 2005, Richardson 2008). Note that NMC guidelines on records and record keeping are under review (NMC 2008).

Record keeping 'is an integral part of the nursing, midwifery and specialist community health nursing practice' (NMC 2005). Records help to make sense of patient care: they communicate information between shifts and between professionals concerning the what, who, why, when and how concerning care provided. Good records not only help to retain information, they also reflect good practice, providing an indication of professionalism, while careless or incomplete record keeping is an indicator of problems with practice (NMC 2005).

NMC (2005) identifies a number of principles that underpin good record keeping. Records should be written in a clear, factual, accurate and consistent style and dated, timed and signed. For legal reasons, records should provide evidence that the duty of care has been discharged through the assessments made, the planning and provision of care, and so on. This applies both to manual records and computer-held records, where the NMC also advises good practice to retain records with reference to the Human Rights Act (2000) and the Caldicott Report (1997). Box 3.1 provides guidelines for good record-keeping.

Box 3.1   Guidelines for Accurate Record Keeping

Accurate Record Keeping

Never alter or falsify a record (credibility is lost if a record is altered or falsified).

In case of errors, draw a line through the error and explain why. Never use correction fluid or a sticker over the error (need to be transparent in what has been documented, maintain credibility and client goals).

Know the trust policy (conveys expectations and any action complies with standards of care).

Document clearly and chronologically the order of care provided (date and time all notations for orderly records).

Record information accurately and completely (provides complete information for all members of the heath care team).

State objectives, factual information and avoid general statements, e.g., 'slept well'.

Sign with name and title legibly (for legal purposes).

Keep records in a safe and confidential manner (to maintain privacy).

(Richardson 2008)

The DH (1997) raised concerns regarding the lack of confidentiality and information security at all levels of the National Health Service (NHS). It pointed out the need to limit access to patient records, including those held on computer, to those who really needed to see them. Healthcare professionals have a common law duty to maintain professional ethical standards of confidentiality. They have a duty to patients, their employer (DH 2002) and their professional body (NMC 2008). Public breaches in confidentiality may result in disciplinary procedures (NMC 2008), while a patient can take legal action over alleged negligence in a 'duty of care' (McHale et al. 1998). The requirement for confidentiality may in certain circumstances be overridden in favour of public interest.

LEARNING ACTIVITY 3.6

You are working in a team that uses shared record-keeping for patients. What are the challenges and potential problems in keeping such records (a) secure, (b) up to date and (c) accurate?

LEARNING ACTIVITY 3.7

Delivering for Health (NHS Scotland 2005: 32) specifies that 'wherever possible clinical staff will record their interventions directly into E-health records, rather than transcribe to written records'. From your practice area, find examples where patient information is recorded electronically.

LEARNING ACTIVITY 3.8

Confidentiality Issues

You are a patient on a ward and have been involved in a serious traffic incident where someone has died. The ward phone rings and a nurse picks it up. It seems someone is asking for you. You hear the nurse saying 'Yes, the patient from the accident is here ... No, I don't think you can speak to them ... Well, they are in quite a serious condition ... Yes, they have a ruptured spleen and have concussion ... Yes, try later .... Goodbye.'

A) Is there anything wrong and if so, what?
B) How should the nurse have handled such a call?

Summary

Nurses need to recognise that communication is a two-way process between sender and receiver. They need too to recognise the potential barriers to effective communication, e.g., language or jargon used, lack of communication skills, cultural beliefs, experiences, assumptions (as first impressions count), perceptual stereotyping (e.g., 'ethnic groups do not speak English'), environment (sitting behind a desk, noise causing a barrier to communication), not listening, sensory loss, jumping to conclusions or patronising people. Nurses must understand how communication is learned and adapt their own communication skills for all individuals and situations, be aware of the barriers to communication and interpersonal skills, and overcome these barriers.

Communication is not an optional extra: it is a core clinical skill vital to nursing care (Wilkinson 1999, Fallowfield et al. 2001). Ineffective communication is associated with emotional burnout, stress and poor job satisfaction (Wilkinson 1994, Ramirez et al. 1995). Effective communication can improve patient satisfaction, compliance and pain control, establish trust and rapport, and support and educate the patient (Fallowfield and Jenkins 1999). As they meet different patients in the course of their work *all* healthcare professionals have regular opportunities to improve their communication skills.

Professional relationships require good communication. It is a prerequisite for building therapeutic relationships with healthcare professionals, patients and their family or carer. Good communication and interpersonal skills in everyday practice provide a basis for effective nursing.

Reflection 1

Ernest Trotter, a 79 year old man, has lived alone since the death of his wife six months ago. The GP surgery has been receiving telephone calls from Ernest's neighbours expressing their concerns about his behaviour – that he has been wandering at night in his pyjamas; watering his garden in the middle of the night; leaving his key in the door; knocking on the neighbour's door looking for his wife.

From your studies and experience to date:

- What factors would you consider might be contributing to his behaviour?
- How would you deal with a situation such as this?
- What communication and interpersonal skills would you use with Ernest to try and ascertain the cause of the situation?

Reflection 2

Adam Smith, a 35 year old man, has suffered from Rheumatoid Arthritis for seven years. He was a fit and active man prior to the onset of his illness and is now confined to a wheelchair. He has been admitted to the ward for reassessment of his drug therapy and pain management. He is extremely knowledgeable about his condition.

On admission Adam is allocated a bed but complains loudly about the fact he is in a bay with five other patients and demands a side room. He is told that there is not one available and he reluctantly unpacks his belongings. Adam ignores the other men in the bay and spends much of his time listening to his MP3 player.

Adam requires help with many of his activities of living but is reluctant to ask for assistance. Adam's wife usually carries out those activities he cannot do independently. Following a moving and handling assessment it is felt that the most appropriate way of transferring Adam is by using the hoist. This is discussed with him but he is adamant that he will not be hoisted. Adam says he would rather remain in bed than be moved in such a demeaning way.

During his stay Adam becomes angry and aggressive towards the staff. He is very direct when care is offered and it can take up to 15 minutes to position Adam so that he is comfortable. The staff are becoming reluctant to interact with Adam and he is frequently allocated to the student nurses to be cared for.

From your studies and experience to date:

- What factors would you consider might attribute to Adam's behaviour?
- What communication and interpersonal skills would you use here with Adam?
- What would you do differently here if anything at all?

Reflection 3

Ben Taylor is a five year old boy who has been admitted to hospital following a road traffic accident. His mother had been collecting Ben from school and was distracted with his younger sister, Lucy, when Ben ran across the road after a friend and was hit by a car. He sustained a fractured femur which is being treated with a skin traction. During this time Ben will be on complete bed rest.

During his initial assessment Ben was distressed and crying so the majority of information was obtained from his mother. He did not want to speak to any of the nurses and kept his eyes closed when the staff asked him a question. However, his mum said that Ben is usually a lively energetic boy who has just started school which he seems to enjoy.

Measurements of Ben's vital signs show that his blood pressure, pulse and respiratory rate are raised but his temperature was normal. His mum states that Ben's normal bedtime was 7.30 pm following a bath and bedtime story read by her and that Ben cannot sleep without his favourite teddy bear.

His mother plans to be resident with Ben and has organised for Lucy to stay with her grandparents. His mother is visibly upset and some of the junior nurses complain to the nurse in charge that she has been verbally aggressive towards them. She blames herself for the accident.

From your studies and experience to date:

- How would you deal with the situation?
- What communication and interpersonal skills would you use here?

References

Ashmore, R (1999) Heron's Intervention Framework: An Introduction and Critique, *Mental Health Nursing* 19(1): 24–27.

Audit Commission (1993) *What Seems to be the Matter: Communication Between Hospitals and Patients.* HMSO, London.

Booth, K et al. (1996) Perceived Professional Support and the Use of Blocking Behaviours by Hospice Nurses, *Journal of Advanced Nursing* 24: 522–527.

Caldicott Report (1997) DH Stationary Office, Norwich

Campbell, S (2006) A Project to Promote Better Communication in Patients, *Nursing Times* 102(19): 28–30.

Chant, S et al. (2001) Communication Skills Training in Healthcare: A Review of the Literature, *Journal of Clinical Nursing* 11: 12–21.

Chant, S et al. (2002) Communication Skills: Some Problems in Nurse Education and Practice, *Journal of Clinical Nursing* 11: 12–21.

DH (1997) *The New NHS: Modern Dependable.* DH, London.

DH (1999) *Making a Difference: Strengthening the Nursing, Midwifery and Health Visiting Contribution to Healthcare.* DH, London.

DH (2000) *Good Practice Guidelines for GP Electronic Records* www.doh.gov/gprep/guidelines.pdf

DH (2002) *Statutory Instrument 2002 No. 1438: The Health Service (Control of Patient Information) Regulations* www.doh.gov.uk/ipv/confiden/instrumement.pdf

Egan, G (2002) *The Skilled Helper A Problem – Management and Opportunity – Development Approach to Helping,* 7th edn. Brook/Cole, Pacific Grove, CA.

ENB (2000) *The Extent to which Educational Programmes Develop the Skills Required to Communicate with People who have Profound Learning and Multiple Disabilities.* ENB, London.

Edwards, M and Davis, H (1997) *Counselling Children with Chronic Medical Conditions.* BPS Books, Leicester.

Fallowfield, L and Jenkins, V (1999) Effective Communication Skills. Are They The Key to Good Cancer Care? *European Journal of Cancer* 35(1): 1592–1597.

Fallowfield, L et al. (2001) Teaching Senior Nurses How to Teach Communication Skills in Oncology, *Cancer Nurse* 24(3): 185–191.

Farrell, G (1996) Telephoning a Nursing Department: Callers' Experience, *Nursing Standard* 10(33): 34–36.

Faugier, J et al. (1997) An Exploration of Clinical Risk Management from a Nursing Perspective, *Nursing Times Research* 2(2): 97–105.

Goldenberg, I and Goldenberg, H (1996) *Family Therapy. An Overview.* Brooks/Cole Publishing, Pacific Grove.

Heaven, C and Maguire, P (1997) Disclosure of Concerns by Hospice Patients and Their Identification by Nurses, *Palliative Medicine* 11(4): 283–290.

Human Rights Act (2000) Home Office, Stationary Office, Norwich.

Lansdown, L (1996) *Children in Hospital.* Oxford University Press, Oxford.

McHale, J et al. (1998) *Law and Nursing.* Butterworth Heinneman, Oxford.

Maguire, P et al. (1996) Helping Cancer Patients Disclose Their Feelings, *European Journal of Cancer Nursing* 32A(1): 78–81.

NHS Scotland (2005) *Delivering for Health. Scottish Executive,* Edinburgh.

NICE (2004) *Improving Supportive and Palliative Care for Adults with Cancer.* NICE, London.

NMC (2004) *Code of Professional Conduct: Standards of Conduct, Performance and Ethics.* NMC, London.

NMC (2005) *Guidelines for Records and Record Keeping.* NMC, London.

NMC (2007) *Guidance for the Introduction of the Essential Skills Cluster for Pre-Registration Nursing Programmes.* NMC, London.

NMC (2008) *A Revolution in Records.* NMC News, London.

Ramirez, AJ et al. (1995) Burnout and Psychiatric Disorder Among Cancer Clinicians, *British Journal of Cancer* 71(6): 1263–1269.

Ravazi, D and Delvaux, N (1997) Communication Skills and Psychological Training in Oncology, *European Journal of Cancer* 33 (6 Supple): S15–S21.

Richardson, R (ed.) (2008) *Clinical Skills for Student Nurses Theory, Practice and Reflection.* Reflect Press, Devon.

Shrubb, D (2001) The Lived Experience of Returning to Healthcare After Instigating Litigation: A Phenomenological Study. Unpublished MSc Dissertation, University of Plymouth.

UKCC (1999) *Fitness for Practice: The UKCC Commission for Nursing and Midwifery Education.* UKCC, London.

UKCC (2000) *Requirements for Pre-Registration Nursing Programmes.* UKCC, London.

Wallace, PR (2001) Improving Palliative Care Through Effective Communication, *International Journal of Palliative Nurse* 7(2): 86–90.

Wilkinson, S (1994) Stress in Cancer Nursing – Does it Really Exist? *Journal of Advanced Nursing* 20(6): 1079–1084.

Wilkinson, S (1999) Communication: It Makes a Difference, *Cancer Nursing* 22(4): 17–20.

www.rnid.org.uk

4

Infection Control and Standard Precautions

Learning Outcomes

This chapter is designed to help you:

o   understand the principles and importance of infection control
o   learn the standard precautions needed
o   understand the importance and role of using personal protective equipment
o   learn how to (a) manage and dispose of waste, (b) deal with spillages, (c) dispose safely of sharps, and (d) handle linen correctly.

Infections and Infection Control

Infections are caused by germs such as **bacteria**, **fungi** or **viruses** entering the body. Well known examples include methicillin resistant staphylococcus aureus (MRSA) and clostridium difficile. The role of hospitals in relation to infection is important. Nightingale (1854) established the principle that 'hospitals should do the sick no harm'. Today, the NMC (2008) requires nurses to work with others to protect and promote the health and wellbeing of those in their care, their families and carers, and the wider community. Consequently, nurses and students need to know the infection control procedures in their practice area.

It has been estimated that 8–10 per cent of patients may acquire a hospital-acquired infection during their stay. The cost to the NHS is at least £1 billion per annum (NPSA 2007). Hospital-acquired (**nosocomial**) infections delay patient recovery, extend the period of hospitalisation, and increase pain, discomfort, anxiety and stress levels. They thereby impact on patients and their families and increase health service costs (Taylor et al. 2001). The Department of Health (2003) acknowledges that healthcare-acquired infections cannot be completely eliminated, but estimates that about one third may be prevented through effective measures (Plowman et al. 1999).

MRSA has become endemic in some hospitals and some senior nurses have suggested that it is out of control (Lines 2006). While rates of patients colonised with MRSA appear to be greater than those infected with MRSA, these infections are significant due to the difficulties in treating systemic infections and the ability of the organism to spread and colonise debilitated patients (Dougherty and Lister 2008). Hand **hygiene** is therefore important in controlling outbreaks of MRSA (Coia et al. 2006). So too is environmental cleanliness as MRSA can survive for long periods in the environment. A prospective microbiological study of MRSA contamination in isolation rooms following the discharge of a MRSA positive patient, found that daily routine cleaning over a four week period did not remove MRSA contamination (Dougherty and Lister 2008). Inadequate cleaning and therefore the removal of exogenous MRSA predisposes to cross-infection with MRSA (Sexton et al. 2006), so once a patient is discharged, the ward must be cleaned thoroughly before the next patient is admitted (Coia et al. 2006).

The transfer of patients with MRSA should be kept to a minimum. The receiving hospital or ward should be given due notification of the patient's arrival, so that the necessary preparation can be made (such as a side room and equipment for the patient). Ambulance and portering staff should also be notified in order to ensure that the ambulance, chair, or bed used to transfer the patient is cleaned before it is used again. In the community, patients colonised with MRSA do not present a risk to healthy people and should live a normal life without any restrictions. In residential homes, strict hand washing, environmental cleanliness and compliance with aseptic technique is required (Coia et al. 2006) when dealing with patients colonised with MRSA.

Clostridium difficile is a slender, gram positive anaerobic rod which is spore forming and motile: it is widely distributed in soil and the intestinal tract of animals (DH 2003a). It can cause foul smelling diarrhoea, abdominal pain and fever. It is found in carpets, blood pressure cuffs, thermometers, nurses' uniforms (DH 2003), radiators, curtain rails, commodes, floors and toilets (Verity et al. 2001). The spores may be transferred when air is disturbed, for example when windows are open or floors are cleaned (Fawley et al. 2005). Clostridium difficile is a common cause of mortality and morbidity in hospitalised patients and has increased in the past several years (Oldfield 2006).

The risk of cross-infection can be reduced by:

- restricting the use of antibiotics that encourage the growth of clostridium difficile
- reducing the duration of antibiotics being administered
- reducing the length of hospitalisation
- careful hand washing
- environmental decontamination
- isolating patients (DH 2003).

Washing hands with detergent and water, drying them carefully and finally cleansing with alcohol hand rub (Boyce et al. 2006) is also required, while cleaning the environment with hypochlorite also reduces the incidence of clostridium difficile (Wilcox et al. 2003).

Infection control must be a priority for nurses across all areas of healthcare, whether in hospital, community, nursing or residential homes. This helps to ensure a safe and clean working environment for staff to work in, ensure that patients receive optimal care and promote health and well-being. Also, all NHS establishments must provide infection control education and training to all clinically based staff as there is a professional obligation for them to develop and maintain the competence, performance, knowledge and skills necessary for safe and effective practice (NMC 2008).

Current national and local infection control policies state that measures must be taken to prevent infections from occurring in healthcare facilities so as to destroy or remove sources of pathogenic **micro-organisms**, thus protecting people from being infected and interrupting the transmission of pathogens. The NICE (2000) clinical guidelines on infection control policies should be followed for any care provided or received at home, in a health centre or clinic, or in the community.

LEARNING ACTIVITY 4.1

From your studies to date answer the following questions.

1   What is a micro-organism?
2   Give two examples of each of the following:

  • bacteria
  • virus
  • fungi

The Health Act (DH 2006) provides basic rules for all NHS organisations to follow when planning and implementing strategies aimed at preventing and controlling healthcare-acquired infections. It sets out criteria for managers of NHS organisations to ensure that patients are cared for in a clean environment and that the risk of healthcare-associated infections is kept as low as possible. The Health Act (DH 2006) works in conjunction with policies such as Health and Safety at Work Act (1974), Management of Health and Safety at Work Regulations (1999), and Health and Safety Executive (2002). The DH (2007, 2008) provides guidance for compliance with these policies, for best practice and evidence-based care.

Community-acquired infections are those acquired outside of healthcare facilities and so already present or incubating at the time of hospital admission. Infection control and prevention in the primary and community settings has tended to be overshadowed by the prominence of such issues within the hospital setting (Judge and Hill 2004). This has been compounded by the disbanding of health authorities and the formation of Primary Care Teams (PCTs) in 2002 and Health Protection Agency (HPA) in 2003: this has raised problems of inconsistency in infection control (Rowland 2006).

To ensure that infection control is consistent, Infection Control Nurses (ICN) need to work alongside those working within the PCT on infection prevention and control. Their roles need to evolve to keep pace with the changing face of healthcare and changes in the significance of various micro-organisms (Perry 2005). The DH (2006a) specifies an infection control infrastructure is required for 'an ICN or other designated person responsible for infection control matters'. This view has been supported by Hughes (2002), who found that the role of the ICN had tended to be shaped by organisational pressures (for example, the prioritisation of risk management, clinical effectiveness and clinical audit).

The NMC (2007) Essential Skills Clusters have emphasised the importance of effective infection control measures, stating that students must be able to 'maintain effective standard infection control precautions for every patient/client'. The DH (2001, 2003, 2004, 2005, 2007) is committed to reducing hospital-acquired infections by establishing standard principles and guidelines regarding infection control for all healthcare practitioners to adhere to when caring for hospital in-patients. The guidelines are grouped into sets of recommendations covering hospital environment, hand hygiene, the use of personal protective equipment and disposal of sharps. The guidelines do not cover the requirements of clinical areas such as the operating department. Box 4.1 highlights the main sites of hospital-acquired infections.

Box 4.1   Sites of Hospital-Acquired Infections

Main Sites of Infection

Urinary	23%
Lower respiratory tract	23%
Surgical wounds	10%
Skin	10%
Blood	6%
Others	28%

(Dougherty and Lister 2008)

Infection control policies and standard precaution methods have never been more important. Whitehouse et al. (2002) estimated that an infection increases the costs of healthcare by more than 300 per cent, emphasising how important it is to prevent infection. Attempts should therefore be made to ensure that hospitalised patients do not acquire infections as patients are indeed susceptible to infections. However, some factors make the prevention of infection either difficult or impossible. These include underlying disease (e.g., chest infection), chronic pulmonary disease, a compromised immune system (as with individuals with HIV) and cancer (where white blood cell production is inhibited). They include too the effect of treatments such as chemotherapy, prescription of antibiotics (which kill resident flora, allowing some strains to multiply) and procedures where the skin is breached (as with **catheters** or intravenous (IV) lines). Patients' age (young and elderly people are particularly susceptible to infection), wounds, the inhalation of airborne particles and hereditary factors can all increase susceptibility to infection.

Healthcare professionals and nurses have a professional obligation to apply infection control measures based on current policy. An example of such a measure would be an audit of current practice of a procedure such as handwashing, together with the education of nurses and doctors to improve practice in the future.

LEARNING ACTIVITY 4.2

Consider your patient group; what factors may place your patients at risk of infection?

Principles of Standard Precautions

Standard precautions as defined by WHO (2006) are the 'simple infection control measures that reduce the risk of transmission of bloodbourne pathogens through exposure to blood or bodily fluids among patients and health care workers'. Standard precautions (sometimes referred to as 'universal precautions' or 'universal control') underpin routine safe practice by protecting staff and patients from infection (RCN 2005). Gammon and Gould (2005) point out that universal precautions are internationally regarded as an effective means of protecting healthcare professionals, patients and the public (for example, the routine use of barrier precautions, in the form of personal protective equipment, to prevent contamination by blood and bodily fluids).

Standard precautions are based on the notion that all blood and bodily fluids are potentially infectious. Thus, standard precautions should be taken with all patients at all times, regardless of whether they are known to have a blood or bodily fluid infection. Standard precautions are applicable to a wide range of situations. They include invasive procedures, the handling of bodily fluids, disposal of clinical waste and sharps, the handling and cleaning of equipment and the disposal of linen.

Standard precautions help to reduce the risk of transmission of pathogens present in blood, bodily fluids, secretions, excretions, skin and mucous membrane. The RCN (2000) has formed a policy dealing with blood and bodily fluids, hand washing, skin abrasions, sharps, protective clothing, spillage and waste. Local trusts should also have their own policies and procedures with regards to the control of infection and the use of standard precautions.

Personal Protective Equipment

Personal protective equipment includes disposable gloves, gowns, aprons, eye protection and masks (Brooker and Waugh 2007). Such equipment is worn if there is a risk of exposure to blood or bodily fluids. They serve to prevent:

- the user's clothing becoming contaminated with pathogenic micro-organisms
- clothing becoming soiled, wet or stained
- the transfer of potential pathogenic micro-organisms from others
- the acquisition of infection from patients (DH 2001, NICE 2003).

However, such equipment can hinder verbal communication. It can also induce anxiety on the part of the patient, who may wonder why the equipment is necessary. It is important to explain to patients why such equipment is worn. In particular, it may be helpful to explain that Health and Safety Executive (1992) regulations require employers to provide employees with appropriate protective equipment such as gloves, while staff have a responsibility to use protective equipment to prevent harm and injury. The decision over whether to use such equipment – and, if so, what level of equipment to use – is based upon a risk assessment of the patient, situation, exposure to healthcare professional's clothing and skin to blood, bodily fluids, secretions or excretions (DH 2001, NICE 2003).

Gloves

Gloves are routinely worn by healthcare professionals to reduce hand contamination by transient pathogens (Kac et al. 2005). The majority of disposable gloves available are made from natural or synthetic latex, or vinyl, and may be in sterile or non-sterile form, either with or without powder. Gloves must conform to Conformite Europeene (CE) standards, be of acceptable quality and available in all clinical areas (DH 2001), should be unpowdered (MDA 1998) and not be made of latex (NHS Executive 1999). The purpose of wearing gloves is to reduce the risk of cross-infection between staff and patient and vice versa (Flores and Pevalin 2006), to act as a barrier, prevent flora from staff being transmitted to patients and reduce transient contamination of the hands of staff by micro-organisms that can be transmitted from patient to another person (ICNA 2002b). Incorrect use of gloves is a common form of poor practice that exposes patients to the risk of cross-infection (Girou et al. 2004). Pratt et al. (2000) and Clark et al. (2002) advise that gloves should not be worn unnecessarily, however, as their prolonged and indiscriminate use may lead to skin sensitivity and adverse reactions. NICE (2003) also advise that any sensitivity or allergy to latex on the part of the patient, carer or healthcare worker should be documented and alternatives be made available.

Pratt et al. (2001) and DH (2005) recommend boxed, clean, non-sterile gloves be worn for routine non-invasive nursing care and when dealing with blood, bodily fluids, secretions, excretions, sharps, contaminated equipment, sterile sites (cannula), aseptic pharmaceutical preparation (chemotherapy) and cleaning (DH 2001). Gloves must be changed between patients and hands washed with bactericidal soap and water or alcohol hand rub (Dougherty and Lister 2008).

Sterile gloves must be worn for surgical aseptic techniques such as the insertion of catheters, wound dressings and surgery (DH 2005). Double-gloving may be used for surgical procedures where gloves become damaged, though double-gloving can cause loss of tactile sensitivity and also increase costs (Dougherty and Lister 2008). Polythene gloves should not be used because they are permeable and are easily damaged, thereby increasing microbial contamination (Pratt et al. 2000, Raybould 2001, Wilson 2001, Clark et al. 2002). Therefore the choice of gloves worn is dependent upon an assessment being made for the task of the risk to the patient and to the healthcare worker (ICNA 2002).

Gloves can become contaminated if:

- the outside of the glove is touched with a bare hand
- anything not sterile is touched while wearing the glove
- the gloved hand falls below waist level
- the glove develops a tear, hole or is punctured.

Gloves are single use items: they must not be cleaned and reused for the same or another patient (NICE 2003). Gloves should be disposed of after contact with patients, when undertaking various procedures on the same patient, when there is a risk of cross contamination, as soon as they become damaged, on completion of a task, or before handling other items (such as a phone or a pen).

It should be emphasised that wearing gloves does not replace the need for hand washing because gloves may be torn and become contaminated. Hand washing is essential both before use and after their removal.

Aprons and gowns

Plastic aprons are frequently worn in hospitals (Callaghan 1998) for protection. They have numerous advantages: they protect the probable area of maximum contamination and are cheap, impervious to moisture and organisms, and easy to put on. They are preferable to cotton gowns, which are readily penetrated by moisture and bacteria (Belkin 2002).

Disposable aprons are worn when the user's own clothing, uniform or skin may become contaminated with micro-organisms. They are also worn when making beds, bathing or toileting patients, dealing with spillages, preparing and serving food, and between patients. Different colour aprons are worn for different tasks: it is important to know the colour code used in your trust.

LEARNING ACTIVITY 4.3

- Identify what types of local protective clothing are available in your local trust.
- How do you think your patients feel about you wearing protective clothing?
- What steps can you take to encourage patients to view the use of protective clothing positively?

Gowns are worn whenever there is a risk of extensive splashing of blood, bodily fluids, secretions or excretions (DH 2001a). This may be in theatres and delivery suites where there is a risk of potential contamination from blood and blood products, bodily fluids, secretions or excretions onto the skin or clothing. Gowns made from Goretex have been introduced to provide protection, to avoid the need for wearing plastic aprons over cotton gowns. Gowns made from Goretex can be laundered, but have the disadvantage of being uncomfortably warm to wear.

Masks

Masks are worn whenever there is a risk of airborne splashing, splattering or spraying into the mouth, nose, or eyes. They must comply with COSHH (HSE 2002) regulations. Masks are worn in theatres to protect the wearer from splashes of blood and bodily fluids onto mucous membranes of the mouth. Close fitting masks or particulate filter personal respiratory protection devices are recommended (DH 2001, Hateley 2003, Health Protection Agency 2004).

However, the wearing of masks for procedures such as wound dressings contributes little to patient or staff safety. Unless the mask fits closely around the mouth and nose, the filtering efficiency of the mask is impaired by wearing the mask for long periods close to the face and moisture collects in the fabric of the mask, thereby interrupting the passage of air through the mask. Micro-organisms can escape from around the edges of the mask (Belkin 1997, Wilson 2001, Leonas and Jones 2003).

Eye Protection

Eye protection is worn where there is a risk of blood splashing onto the face, when sterilising and disinfecting endoscopes and other surgical equipment with chemicals (Mangram et al. 1999, Pearson 2000, DH 2001, Wilson 2001). Protection includes face shields, spectacles, goggles or visors and are worn in theatres (Keogh et al. 2001), obstetrical procedures, barrier nursing (Parker and Goldman 2006), dentistry and endoscopy. They must be optically clear (scratch and mark-free), anti-fog and distortion-free, close fitting and shielded at the sides. They may be reusable after cleaning or for single use only.

Hats

Unless there is heavy contamination or splashing, wearing a hat is not justified. Clean and tidy hair has not been implicated in cross infection and hence there is no need to wear hats when nursing infected patients. Hats are only worn in theatre for infection control purposes (Mangram et al. 1999): they have been shown to reduce wound infections (Friberg et al. 2001).

Protective Footwear

Floors on hospital wards easily become contaminated by large numbers of bacteria (Ayliffe et al. 2000). However, there is no evidence that the use of overshoes reduces bacterial counts on theatre floors (Weightman and Banfield 1994). While washable shoes must be available for those entering the operating theatre (Ayliffe et al. 2000), footwear worn elsewhere in the hospital should be chosen to comply with risk management, rather than for infection control reasons.

There is no evidence to show that shoe coverings reduce contamination of clean floors (Santos et al. 2005). Shoe coverings should be used when there is contamination of the environment, as part of COSHH requirements (HSE 2002a). The only established link to an infection was an outbreak of pseudomonas on the hands of staff in a renal unit when they were putting on the overshoes (Ayliffe et al. 1999).

Waste Management and Disposal

Most waste goes to landfill or incineration or is disposed of using alternative technologies (RCN 2007). Irrespective of the method of disposal, waste has the potential to pollute land, air and water. Managing healthcare waste is therefore a crucial part of infection control. There is a statutory requirement for healthcare facilities to comply with local, national and international regulations and legislation relating to the segregation, handling, transportation and disposal of waste. Examples of regulation or legislation include COSHH Carriage of Dangerous Goods (Classification, Packaging and Labelling) and Use of Tansportable Pressure Receptacles Regulations (DH 2004), Safe Management of Healthcare Waste 2006 (DH 2006a), the Health Services Advisory Committee (1999) and Occupational Safety and Health Administration (2004).

The RCN (2007) states that most healthcare waste (between 75–90 per cent) is similar to domestic waste (e.g., paper or packaging), while 10–15 per cent is infectious or hazardous waste that poses a risk to human health or the environment. In the event of a failure to separate the two, all waste must be treated as infectious waste. Due to regulatory changes including Landfill Regulations, Hazardous Waste Regulations and List of Waste Regulations, all healthcare waste must now be classified using the European Waste Catalogue (EWC) codes. In Scotland, the List of Waste Regulations doesn't apply, as 'hazardous waste' is defined as 'special waste' under Special Waste Regulations. Sharps or medicinal products may be placed in a landfill in a permitted or licensed site. Recyclable components should be segregated while clear or opaque receptacles can be used for domestic waste.

The management of clinical waste is regulated by DH (2006c). There have been a number of key changes. These include the removal of the 'clinical waste groups A to E' definitions and the introduction of new identification terms (e.g., healthcare waste, infectious waste, medicinal waste, offensive/hygiene waste). There is also a revised colour-coding system for the disposal of waste. A unified approach to segregating waste is the 'colour-coded scheme' used to ensure standardisation across the UK (see Box 4.2).

Box 4.2   Colour-Coded Scheme for Disposal of Waste

Colour	Description
Yellow	Infectious waste requiring incineration, e.g., anatomical waste, radioactive waste
Orange	Infectious waste which can be incinerated
Purple	**Cytotoxic** and **cytostatic** waste must be incinerated in a permitted or licensed facility, e.g., colour-coded sharps, infectious waste
Yellow/Black	Offensive/hygiene waste which may be placed in a landfill in a permitted or licensed site
Black	Domestic waste not containing infectious waste

(RCN 2007)

There are two types of healthcare waste – hazardous and non-hazardous as identified in Box 4.3.

Box 4.3   Types of Healthcare Waste

Hazardous Waste	Non-Hazardous Waste
Infectious waste, e.g., anatomical waste, sharps	Offensive/hygiene waste, e.g., incontinence pads and other human hygiene, sanitary waste, nappies
Cytotoxic and cytostatic medicines	Non-cytotoxic and non-cytostatic medicines, e.g., controlled drugs should be referred to the appropriately authorised personnel for disposal and destruction
Healthcare chemicals and hazardous properties	Domestic waste
Batteries	Packaging waste
X-ray photochemicals	Recyclable materials
Radioactive waste	Food waste

(RCN 2007)

The RCN (2007) acknowledges the complexities surrounding the removal of clinical waste in community settings. It specifies two options: securely carrying the waste in rigid, air-tight packages from the patient's home to base, where the waste can be collected and disposed of appropriately (though with risk, through moving and handling, of cross-contamination (McCulloch 1998)); or have the waste collected from the patient's home by an approved waste contractor, local authority or health provider. Colour-coded waste packaging still applies here as noted in Box 4.4.

Box 4.4   Colour-Coded Waste Packaging

Colour	Rationale
Orange	Used for products that can be rendered safe, e.g., dressings, bandages, some plastic single use instruments
Yellow	Contains waste products for incineration, e.g., anatomical waste (placenta)
Yellow/Purple	Waste contaminated with cytotoxic and cytostatic medicinal products, e.g., chemotherapy, antiviral and/or hormonal drugs
Yellow/Black	Non-infectious or non-hazardous waste
Black	Domestic waste

(RCN 2007)

Cyto medicines and all associated sharps and liquid residues should be disposed of in a sharps container with a purple lid. In all other cases it is acceptable to use containers with a yellow lid. The RCN (2007) recognises that, for practical reasons, community nurses may wish to use one sharps container and if so, a container with a purple lid should be used. Infected or contaminated plastic disposable instruments containing no risk of sharps may be disposed of as infectious waste in the orange bag. Contaminated metal disposable instruments containing no risk of sharps may be disposed of in a rigid yellow container marked 'For incineration only'. Most non-infectious instruments containing no risk of sharps may be disposed of as 'offensive/hygiene' waste and in the case of metal instruments may be reclaimed and recovered, where available (RCN 2007).

LEARNING ACTIVITY 4.4

Consider how waste is disposed of in your practice area.

- Identify what constitutes:
  - clinical
  - household
  - sharps waste.
- Who else, besides you, is involved in waste disposal?

Managing Spillages

Spillages should be dealt with immediately in accordance with local policy. Wherever spillage has occurred, it should be disinfected properly. The policy should specify reporting and investigation procedures, safe systems of work for cleaning up the spillage, appropriate requirements for decontamination and personal protective equipment to be worn (RCN 2007).

REFER TO PROCEDURE: SPILLAGES

Disposal of Sharps

'Sharps' refer to any sharp instrument or object used in the delivery of healthcare that might cut, graze or prick. They include needles, suture needles, scalpel blades, lancets, stitch cutters, contaminated broken glass and intravenous cannulae. Injuries often occur when recapping hypodermic needles after use or manipulating used sharps (for example, bending, breaking or cutting hypodermic needles), when sharp items are discovered in an unexpected area (e.g., in a bed), or when a client moves suddenly (perhaps when an injection is being administered). The item used must be disposed of in a colour-coded sharps container: the colour is defined by the waste it contains and is treated and disposed of as noted in Box 4.5.

Box 4.5   Colour-Coded Sharps Container

Colour of Lid	Rationale
Orange	Not contaminated with medicinal product or contaminated with medicinal products other than cyto-medicines
Yellow	Undischarged sharp or syringe partially discharged is contaminated with residual medicine Container is incinerated
Purple	Contaminated with cytotoxic and cytostatic medicinal products Must be incinerated

(RCN 2007)

To reduce the risk of injury and exposure to blood-borne viruses, used sharps must be discarded in accordance with DH (2006b) guidelines. These specify that the sharps container must be available at the point of use. The user must dispose of the sharps themselves, not remove the needle from the syringe before its disposal, never re-sheath, break, bend or manipulate the needle, and never pass sharps directly from hand to hand. They must keep handling to a minimum (NICE 2003).

The sharps container should conform to UN3291 and BS7320 standards or equivalent. It must be located in a safe position, not on the floor. It must be disposed of when three quarters full (there should be a 'Do not fill above this line' warning). When a container is to be disposed of, it should be closed, labelled with details of the ward and hospital name, dated and sent for incineration. Sharps containers must never be left on the floor in public areas (DH 2001, NICE 2003).

Linen

Used linen is potentially an infection risk for all those who are involved in its handling. This is especially so if the linen is contaminated with body substances, or has been used in the care of patients with infectious diseases. Linen is laundered between patient use, and when visibly soiled, in order to reduce microbial counts. This produces a negligible infection risk. To prevent cross-infection from linen, wear gloves and an apron, avoid shaking linen (so micro-organisms will not be dispersed) and ensure that it is washed at 70 degrees centigrade minimum in order to destroy micro-organisms. Soiled linen from patients with blood-borne viruses or tuberculosis should be placed in water soluble plastic bags with a red soluble outer bag before being transported to laundry for washing. Contaminated linen must be placed immediately in the linen, not placed temporarily elsewhere. The skip should only be filled to three quarters full. Place the linen skip close to the bed and ensure that all sharps are discarded before the linen is discarded.

LEARNING ACTIVITY 4.5

A local hospital has it own laundry department which routinely collects and delivers clean linen to the various wards within the hospital. It is common practice for the laundry employees to use bare hands to collect the dirty laundry since it is stored in plastic bags. The employees then assess how much clean linen is needed and leaves sufficient linen before moving to the next ward.

- Is this appropriate practice?
- If not, why?

Summary

Infection control and standard precautions are an essential part of healthcare practice. It is needed to ensure safety of staff, patients and the wider community. Everyone involved in providing care in the community should be educated about standard procedures and trained in hand decontamination, use of protective clothing and safe disposal of sharps. Nurses need to keep up to date with current research findings on infection control. Healthcare professionals have a legal and ethical duty of care to promote an ethos that reduces the risk of infection within the healthcare environment (Portsmouth 2007).

LEARNING ACTIVITY 4.6

A patient has been admitted to your ward suffering from diarrhoea and vomiting. Viral gastroenteritis is suspected.

A)   What risk factors indicate that the patient is an infection risk to others?
B)   What protective clothing should be available for staff to wear?

PROCEDURE: SPILLAGES

- Wear gloves and an apron when cleaning the spillage
- Clean the surface(s) contaminated with bodily fluid with a solution of household bleach in water (1 part bleach to 10 parts water)
- Take care to avoid contact between the solution and exposed skin or clothing
- Dispose of all swabs, dressings, gloves and apron into clinical waste bag
- Wash hands immediately after cleaning the spillage as per local policy.

PROCEDURE: BLOOD AND BODILY FLUID SPILLAGES

- Remove all spills of blood or bodily fluid immediately, following local policy
- Use appropriate disinfectant to neutralise the spill, e.g., sodium hypochlorite (except for urine spillage) 1 per cent or 10, 000 ppm of available chlorine because organic material rapidly inactivates chlorine and results in irritation. Clear soluble phenolics, peroxygen or quaternary ammonia compounds may be used instead. However, refer to local policy and Infection Control Teams for advice
- Wear protective clothing, e.g., gloves, an apron and use clear signs
- Wash hands immediately after cleaning the spillage and dispose of gloves and apron into waste bag
- Clothing soiled by bodily fluids should be washed using a hot cycle wash as the heat kills any viruses present.

PROCEDURE: SPILLAGES VISIBLY CONTAMINATED WITH BLOOD

- Sprinkle chlorine releasing granules over the spillage to cover and soak up the blood
- Leave for up to 5 minutes
- While wearing gloves and an apron wipe up the spillage with paper towels and dispose into clinical waste bag
- Clean the surface(s) using detergent and water
- Remove and dispose of gloves and apron into clinical waste bag
- Wash hands immediately as per local policy.

PROCEDURE: URINE SPILLAGES VISIBLY CONTAMINATED WITH BLOOD

- Soak up the urine as thoroughly as possible with paper towels
- Clean the areas with detergent and water while wearing gloves and an apron
- If necessary use chlorine agent to disinfect the areas (but be aware of any irritation that may occur)
- Place waste material into clinical waste bag with gloves and apron
- Wash hands immediately as per local policy.

PROCEDURE: SPILLAGES OF BODILY FLUIDS (FAECES, URINE, VOMIT) NOT VISIBLY CONTAMINATED WITH BLOOD

- Soak up the spillage with paper towels
- Discard the paper towels and any other waste from the spillage into clinical waste bag while wearing gloves and an apron
- Clean the area with detergent and water
- Discard gloves and apron into clinical waste bag
- Wash hands immediately as per local policy.

PROCEDURE: MERCURY SPILLAGES

- Where mercury is used a risk assessment and written procedures are required and followed. A mercury spillage kit should be used containing the following:

  - disposable gloves
  - paper towels
  - bulb aspirator (to collect large drops of mercury)
  - vapour mask
  - receptacle fitted with a seal
  - mercury absorbent paste.

References

Ayliffe, GAJ et al. (1999) *Hospital Acquired Infection: Principles and Practice,* 3rd edn. Butterworth Heinneman, Oxford.

Ayliffe, GAJ et al. (2000) *Control of Hospital Infection: A Practical Handbook,* 4th edn. Arnold, London.

Belkin, NL (1997) The Evolution of the Surgical Mask: Filtering Efficiency versus Effectiveness, *Journal of Infection Control and Hospital Epidemiology* 18(1): 4–56.

Belkin, NL (2002) A Historical Review of Barrier Material, *AORN J* 76(4): 648–653.

Boyce, JM et al. (2006) Lack of Association Between the Increased Incidence of Clostridium Difficile Associated Diseases and the Increasing Use of Alcohol Based Handrub, *Journal of Hospital Infection* 34: 191–196.

Brooker, C and Waugh, A (2007) *Foundations of Nursing Practice. Fundamentals of Hospital Care.* Mosby, Edinburgh.

Callaghan, I (1998) Bacterial Contamination of Nurses Uniforms: A Study, *Nursing Standard* 13(1): 37–42.

Clarke, L et al. (2002) *Protective Clothing: Principles and Guidance.* Infection Control Nurses Association, London.

Coia, JE et al. (2006) Guidelines for the Control and Prevention of Methicillin – Resistant Staphylococcus Aureus (MRSA) in Healthcare Facilities by the Joint BSAC/HIS/ICNA Working Party on MRSA, *Journal of Hospital Infection* 63 (Suppl), S1–S44

DH (2001) Standard Principles for Preventing Hospital Acquired Infections, *Journal of Hospital Infection* 47 (Suppl): S21–S37.

DH (2001a) Standard Principles for Preventing Hospital-Acquired Infections, *Journal of Hospital Infection* 47(Suppl): S21–S37.

DH (2003) *Winning Ways: Working Together to Reduce Healthcare Associated Infections in England.* DH, London.

DH (2003a) *National Clostridium Difficile Standards Group Report to the Department of Health Feb 2003.* DH, London.

DH (2004) *Towards Cleaner Hospitals and Lower Rates of Infection: A Summary of Action.* DH, London.

DH (2005) *Saving Lives: A Delivery Programme to Reduce Healthcare Associated Infection (HCAI) Including MRSA.* DH, London.

DH (2006) *The Health Act 2006 Code of Practice for the Prevention and Control of Healthcare Acquired Infection* www.dh.gov.uk

DH (2006a) *Saving Lives: A Delivery Programme to Reduce Healthcare Associated Infections.* DH, London.

DH (2006b) *Code of Practice for the Prevention and Control of the Healthcare Associated Infections.* DH, London.

DH (2006c) *Health Technical Memorandum 07–01: Safe Management of Health Care Waste.* The Stationary Office, London.

DH (2007) *Essential Steps to Safe, Clean Care: Reducing Healthcare Associated Infections.* DH, London.

DH (2008) *Clean, Safe Care – Reducing Infections and Saving Lives.* DH, London.

Dougherty, L and Lister, S (2008) *The Royal Marsden Hospital Manual of Clinical Nursing Procedures Student Edition,* 7th edn. Wiley Blackwell, Oxford.

Fawley, WN et al. (2005) Molecular Epidemiology of Endemic Clostridium Difficile Significance of Subtypes of the UK Epidemic (Ribotype 1), *Journal of Clinical Microbiology* 43(6): 2685–2696.

Flores, A and Pevalin, DJ (2006) Healthcare Workers' Knowledge and Attitudes to Glove Use, *British Journal of Infection Control* 7(5): 18–22.

Friberg, B et al. (2001) Surgical Area Contamination Comparable Bacterial Counts Using Disposable Head and Mask and Helmet Aspirator System, But Dramatic Increase Upon Omission of Head Gear: An Experimental Study in Horizontal Laminar Airflow, *Journal of Hospital Infection* 47(2): 110–115.

Gammon, J and Gould, D (2005) Universal Precautions: A Review of Knowledge Compliance and Strategies to Improve Practice, *Journal of Research Nursing* 10(5): 529–547.

Girou, E et al. (2004) Misuse of Gloves: The Foundation for Poor Compliance with Hand Hygiene and Potential for Microbial Transmission, *Journal of Hospital Infection* 57(2): 162–169.

Hateley, P (2003) Infection Control. In Brooker C and Nichol M (eds) *Nursing Adults: The Practice of Caring.* Mosby, Edinburgh.

Health Protection Agency (2004) Information on Face Masks and Respirators www.hps.org.uk/infections/topics_az/SARS/maskFAQ.htm

Health Service Advisory Committee (1999) *Safe Disposal of Clinical Waste.* HMSO, London.

Health and Safety Executive (1992) *Personal Protective Equipment at Work Regulations: Guidance on Regulations.* HMSO, London.

Health and Safety Executive (2002) Control of Substances Hazardous to Health Regulations: A Brief Guide to the Regulations. What You Need to Know about Control of Substances Hazardous to Health Regulations www.hse.gov.uk

HSE (2002a) *Control of Substances Hazardous to Health (COSHH) Approved Code of Practice.* HSE, London.

Health and Safety at Work Act (1974). HMSO, London.

Hughes, S (2002) The Role of the Nurse Consultant in Infection Control, *British Journal of Infection Control* 3(5): 26–29.

ICNA (2002) *A Comprehensive Glove Choice*. ICNA, Bathgate.

ICNA (2002a) *Protective Clothing: Principles and Guidance*. Lance Publishing, Fitwise Bathgate.

Infection A2Z (2005) Decontamination Processes Disinfection www.healthcarea2z.org

Judge, C and Hill, D (2004) Developing Infection Control Services Within Primary Care, *British Journal of Infection Control* 5: 20–22.

Kac, G et al. (2005) Microbiological Evaluation of Second Hand Hygiene Procedures Achieved by Healthcare Workers During Routine Patients Care: A Randomised Study, *Journal of Hospital Infection* 60(1). 32 39.

Keogh, IJ et al. (2001) Blood Splash and Tonsillectomy: An Underestimated Hazard to the Otolaryngologist, *Journal of Laryngol Otol* 115(6): 455–456.

Leonas, KK and Jones, CR (2003) The Relationship of Fabric Properties and Bacterial Filtering Efficiency for Selected Surgical Masks, *Journal of Textile and Apparel Technology and Management* 3(2): 1–8.

Lines, J (2006) A Study of Senior Nurses Perception About MRSA, *Nursing Times* 102(15): 32–35.

Management of Health and Safety at Work Regulations (1999). In St John Holt A (2002) *Principles of Health and Safety at Work,* 6th edn. IOSH Services, Leicestershire.

Mangram, AJ et al. (1999) Guidelines for Prevention of Surgical Sire Infection, *American Journal of Infection Control* 27(2): 97–134.

McCulloch, J (1998) Infection Control: Principles for Practice, *Nursing Standard* 13(1): 49–53, 55–56.

MDA (1998) *Latex Medical Gloves*. DH, London.

NHS Executive (1999) *Variant Creutzfeldt-Jakob Disease (vCJD) Minimising the Risk of Transmission*. DH, London.

NICE (2000) *Infection Control Prevention of Hospital Acquired Infections in Primary and Community Care*. NICE, London.

NICE (2003) *Infection Control: Prevention of Healthcare – Associated Infections in Primary and Community Care,* (No. 1). Standard Principles NICE, London.

Nightingale, F (1854) *Notes on Nursing: What It Is and What It Is Not*. Harrison, London.

NPSA (2007) Home Page www.npsa.nhs.uk/cleanyourhands/the-campaign/background

NMC (2007) *Guidance for the Introduction of the Essential Skills Clusters for Pre-Registration Nursing Programmes*. NMC, London.

NMC (2008) *The Code: Standards, Performance and Ethics for Nurses and Midwives*. NMC, London.

Occupational Safety and Health Administration (2004) TB: Healthcare Wide Hazards Module www.osha.gov

Oldfield, EC (2006) C Difficile Associated Diarrhoea: Resurgence with a Vengence, *Rev Gastroenteraol Disord* 6(2): 79–96.

Parker, MJ and Goldman RD (2006) Paediatric Emergency Department Staff Perceptions of Infection Control Measures Against Server Acute Resp Syndrome, *Emergency Medicine Journal* 23(5): 349–353.

Pearson, T (2000) The Wearing of Facial Protection in High Risk Environments, *British Journal of Perioperative Nursing* 10(3): 163–166.

Perry, C (2005) The Infection Control Nurse in England – Past, Present and Future, *British Journal of Infection Control* 6(5): 18–21.

Plowman, R et al. (1999) *The Socio-Economic Burden of Hospital Acquired Infections*. Public Health Laboratory Service, London.

Portsmouth, J (2007) Infection Control and the Law: Legal and Ethical Obligations, *British Journal of Infection Control* 8(2): 14–19.

Pratt, RJ et al. (2000) *Epic Phase 1: The Development of National Evidence Based Guidelines for Preventing Hospital Acquired Infections in England Standard Principles: Technical Report*. Thames Valley University, London.

Pratt, RJ et al. (2001) The Epic Project: Developing National Evidence-Based Guidelines for Preventing Healthcare Associated Infections, *Journal of Hospital Infection* 47(2): S1–S82.

Raybould, LM (2001) Disposable Non Sterile Gloves: A Policy for Appropriate Usage, *British Journal of Nursing* 10(17): 1135–1141.

Rowland, D (2006) *Mapping Communicable Disease Control Administration in the UK: Between Devolution and Europe*. Nuffield Trust, London.

RCN (2000) *Universal Precautions for the Control of Infection*. RCN, London.

RCN (2005) *Good Practice in Infection Prevention and Control. Guidance for Nursing Staff*. RCN, London.

RCN (2007) *Safe Management of Health Care Waste*. RCN Guidance, London.

Santos, AM et al. (2005) Evidence of Control and Prevention of Surgical Site Infection by Shoe Cover and Private Shoes: A Systematic Literature Review, *Rev Lat Am Enfermagen* 13(1): 86–92.

Scottish Statutory Instrument (2003) *The Landfill (Scotland) Regulations*. The Stationary Office, Edinburgh.

Scottish Statutory Instrument (2004) *Special Waste Amendment (Scotland) Regulations*. The Stationary Office, Edinburgh.

Sexton, T et al. (2006) Environmental Reservoirs of MRSA in Invasive Human Disease *BMC Microbiology* 6(1): 67.

Statutory Instrument (2002) *The Landfill (England and Wales) Regulations*. The Stationary Office, London.

Statutory Instrument (2005) *The Hazardous Waste (England and Wales) Regulations*. The Stationary Office, London.

Statutory Rule (2003) *The Landfill Regulations (NI)*. The Stationary Office, Belfast.

Statutory Rule (2005) *The Hazardous Waste Regulations (NI)*. The Stationary Office, Belfast.

Taylor, K et al. (2001) *The Challenge of Hospital Acquired Infections*. NAO, London.

Verity, P et al. (2001) Prospective Evaluation of Environmental Contamination by C. difficile in Isolation Side Rooms, *Journal of Hospital Infection* 49(3): 204–209.

Weightman, NC and Banfield, KR (1994) Protective Overshoes are Unncessary in a Day Surgery Unit, *Journal of Hospital Infection* 28: 1–3.

Whitehouse, JD et al. (2002) The Impact of Surgical – Site Infections following Orthopaedic Surgery at a Community and a University Hospital: Adverse Quality of Life, Excess Length of Stay and Extra Cost, *Infect Control Hosp Epidemiol* 23(4): 183–189.

Wilcox, MH et al. (2003) Comparison of the Effect of Detergent Versus Hypochlorite Cleaning on Environmental Contamination and Incidence of C. Difficile, *Journal of Hospital Infection* 54(2): 109–114.

Wilson, J (2001) *Infection Control in Clinical Practice,* 2nd edn. Balliere Tindall, Edinburgh.

WHO (2006) Universal Precautions Including Injections Safety www.who.int/hiv/topics/precautions/universalen/print www.medical-devices.gov.uk/mda

5

Hand Washing and Aseptic Technique

Learning Outcomes

This chapter is designed to help you:

o   understand the importance of hand washing
o   learn the principles of hand washing
o   understand the importance of aseptic technique
o   learn the principles of aseptic technique.

Introduction

Patients expect to be protected from acquiring an infection, while nurses have a professional responsibility and duty of care to protect their patient's well being (King 1998, NMC 2008). Hand washing and aseptic technique play an important role in ensuring these ideals are met.

The Importance of Hand Washing

Hand washing is the most important procedure for preventing nosocomial infections. Hands have been shown to be an important route of transmission of infection (DH 2001, Pittet and Boyce 2001). Gould et al. (2007) and Lugg and Ahmed (2008) confirm that hand decontamination is the most important measure for preventing the transmission of infections. International studies have shown that infection rates can be reduced by 10–50 per cent simply by cleaning hands (Pittet et al. 2000, NHSQIS 2005, RCN 2005). This can significantly reduce infection rates in gastrointestinal infections, intensive care units, methicillin sensitive staphylococcus aureus (MSSA) and methicillin resistant staphylococcus aureus (MRSA). However, evidence suggests that many healthcare professionals do not decontaminate their hands as often as they need to, nor use the correct technique (RCN 2005).

Both the WHO (2005) 'Clean Hospital, Clean Healthcare' programme and DH (2005) 'Wash Your Hands' campaign emphasised the key role of hand washing. Hand washing has tended to be an undervalued activity. Burnett et al. (2008) found that patient hand hygiene received only limited recognition in the control and prevention of hospital-acquired infection. The purpose of hand washing is to remove pathogenic micro-organisms (whether transient or resident) from the skin.

You must decontaminate your hands after performing any activity that may contaminate your hands and before direct contact with any patient or site on a patient. Hands should be washed whenever dealing with bodily fluids, caring for people in isolation, before and after wearing protective equipment, handling food or medication, or when one is involved with patient care.

Hands that have been washed but have not been dried well can transfer micro-organisms. In fact, they may do so more easily than dry hands as damp hands contain greater numbers of micro-organisms (Patrick et al. 1997, Gould 2000, Taylor et al. 2000), while inadequately dried hands are prone to skin damage (RCN 2005). Paper towels are a quick, thorough and effective means for hand drying, though disliked due to roughness (Gould 1994, Redway et al. 1994, Ward 2000). Cloth towels are slightly more effective in removing bacteria (Blakemore and Proski 1984). Warm air dryers are the least effective method of hand drying: they are noisy, they take longer to dry hands, they can be used by only one person at a time, they may fan bacteria into the atmosphere and recontaminate the hands. Knight et al. (1993) and Redway et al. (1994) have suggested that warm air dryers increase bacteria count by over 50 per cent and increase bacterial contamination of the local environment. Yamamoto et al. (2005) note that air drying or disposable paper towels are the usual methods of hand drying: bacterial counts on palms and hands increase after being dried using warm air driers. Paper towels are the most useful method for removing bacteria from fingertips.

Patients have a right to be protected from preventable infections. NPSA (2004a) indicated that patients want to be involved in helping to improve hand hygiene, while a National Audit Office (2004) report encouraged active public participation in measures to improve staff and visitor compliance with good infection and control practice.

Nurses therefore need to ensure that all healthcare professionals wash their hands on all occasions (and also wear protective clothing when in contact with infectious material or those in isolation). The intention is to prevent cross-infection to other patients and protect health providers, thereby minimising the risk of infection being spread. However, studies have shown poor hand hygiene compliance following inappropriate glove use. This finding was supported by Pittet et al. (2000), who found that healthcare workers were less likely to wash their hands after wearing gloves. Pittet et al. (2004) found that while 85 per cent of physicians perceived hand hygiene to be important in minimising the risk of cross transmission between patients, only 57 per cent actually adhered to hand hygiene procedures. Girou et al. (2004) found hand hygiene was not performed (due to improper gloving) in 64.4 per cent of instances. Failure to remove contaminated gloves was a major component in poor compliance with hand hygiene and carried a high risk of microbial transmission, while an observational study by Whitby and McLaws (2004) found glove use diminished compliance with hand washing protocols. Therefore, hand washing should be strongly encouraged after glove removal (Pittet and Boyce 2001). Failure to do so constitutes non-compliance with hand hygiene recommendations (Pittet and Boyce 2001).

LEARNING ACTIVITY 5.1

In your clinical area:

- What facilities are available for the healthcare professionals to wash and dry their hands?
- What other provisions are there for healthcare professionals to wash and dry their hands?
- How frequently do the healthcare professionals wash and dry their hands?

Hands must be washed whenever there is a chance they may have become contaminated or whenever there is a risk of transmitting infection to others (patients, practitioners, visitors and friends).

There are three types of hand washing, each with its own purpose. Table 5.1 identifies the solutions used and reasons for their use. The first type is social hand washing. This involves using soap and water for between 10–15 seconds, with rinsing in running water effectively to remove visibly soiled dirt, organic material and transient micro-organisms from the skin. (As some bacteria grow on bars of soap especially if wet, use dry or use liquid soap dispensers.)

Second, there is aseptic hand washing. This involves using antiseptic preparations, for example chlorhexidine, triclosan, provodine-iodine. It not only removes dirt and transient flora from the skin, but also kills or inhibits the growth of resident micro-organisms. Some preparations work for several hours after their initial use and are useful in high risk situations (e.g., invasive procedures, caring for patients in isolation). Antiseptics used on the skin are not suitable for hard surfaces and should not be used to clean equipment.

Third, alcohol-based hand rubs (containing 70 per cent alcohol and emollients that act rapidly and kill or inhibit the growth of transient and resident micro-organisms) are an acceptable alternative to hand washing, though ineffective if the hands are visibly soiled with dirt, blood or other material, as alcohol does not remove dirt).

ICNA (2007) advises that routine hand washing using soap and water or an alcohol-based preparation is adequate for most clinical activities, while the International Federation of Infection Control (IFIC) states that antiseptic or alcohol-based preparation should be used for hand washing at the following times:

- before and after nursing a patient
- before performing an invasive procedure
- before caring for a patient who is more susceptible to infections, e.g., neonate, immunocompromised
- before and after touching a wound, catheter or other in-dwelling device
- before and after wearing gloves
- after contact with blood or bodily fluids
- following any activity where contamination is likely to occur
- after contact with someone with a transmissible pathogen, e.g., MRSA.

Applying alcohol-based hand rubs to hands is a fast, simple and effective method of reducing micro-organisms present on hands. The use of rubs can improve hand hygiene compliance and reduce the risk of transmission of infection in healthcare, but the hands should be free from dirt and organic material when used (NICE 2003). Alcohol hand gel must be available at the 'point of care' in all primary and secondary care settings (NPSA 2004). Frequent use of alcohol products can dry the skin unless an emollient ingredient is included in the formulation.

Table 5.1 *Solutions used for hand washing*

Indications for Use	Soap	Antiseptic Preparations	Alcohol Rub
Removes transient micro-organisms	X	X	X
Removes resident micro-organisms		X	X
Effective on physically soiled hands	X	X	X
Routine use in clinical areas	X	X	X
Suitable for pre-operative preparation		X	X
Hand preparation before invasive preparation		X	X

(Wilson 2001)

In laboratory conditions alcohol gel was found to kill 99 per cent of pathogens, including MRSA (Brighton and Sussex University Hospital 2003, Hugonnet and Pittet 2000). It does not eradicate clostridium difficile and thus trolleys and other equipment should not be washed with alcohol-based hand rubs. Instead, such equipment should be cleaned daily and when contaminated cleaned with a detergent solution, and dried carefully with paper towels. This will remove a high proportion of micro-organisms including bacterial spores (Ayliffe et al. 2000).

Principles of Hand Washing

The principles of good hand hygiene require: an understanding of why hands need to be washed, selection of the correct cleansing product (social, aseptic, alcohol rub); and correct preparation and technique. Fingernails need to be kept short, rings and wristwatches should not be worn; long sleeves should be rolled up; hands should be rinsed and dried properly; and false fingernails should not be worn (Colombo et al. 2002, Porteus 2002).

An effective hand washing technique includes three stages: preparation; washing and rinsing; and drying. The most important factors preventing hand washing include lack of education, high workload, lack of a role model from key staff and lack of administrative leadership (Pittet and Boyce 2001), poorly accessed sinks, an insufficient supply of hand rubs, skin problems (e.g., psoriasis), the negative influence of colleagues, hand washing being given a low priority generally, or lack of motivation (Storr and Clayton 2004).

REFER TO PROCEDURE: HAND WASHING

Principles of Asepsis/Aseptic Technique

Xavier (1999: 49–53) defines **asepsis** as 'the prevention of microbial contamination of living tissue or fluid or sterile materials by excluding, removing or killing micro-organisms'. Asepsis can be divided into two types – (1) medical or clean asepsis which tries to reduce the number of organisms to a specific area, thereby limiting their spread, and (2) surgical or sterile asepsis (Ayliffe et al. 2000), which includes procedures to eliminate micro-organisms from areas such as theatres or treatment rooms.

Aseptic technique is the practice implemented to prevent the risk of infection (Dougherty and Lister 2008). The aim is to protect the patient from contamination by pathogenic organisms during medical and nursing procedures, and to protect healthcare workers from being exposed to potential infected blood and bodily fluids. The aim of aseptic technique is to prevent micro-organisms on hands, equipment and surfaces from being introduced to susceptible body sites (Wilson 2001, Burton and Englekirk 2004). There are two aims of aseptic technique – protecting the patient from contamination by pathogenic organisms during procedures and protecting the healthcare worker from being exposed to potential infectious blood and bodily fluids (Dougherty and Lister 2008). This is achieved by ensuring that only sterile equipment and fluids are used. Aseptic technique is often referred to as the 'non-touch' technique, ensuring that hands do not contaminate sterile equipment or the patient by using forceps or sterile gloves (DH 2001). Forceps, however, can damage skin tissue, while gloves can become contaminated or damaged during use (David 1991, Driever et al. 2001, Kocent et al. 2002, Kelsall et al. 2006). A poor aseptic technique can result in contamination; with effective risk assessment and management (Chalmers and Straub 2006) infections can be prevented and controlled.

Bree-Williams and Waterman (1996) found that not all nurses followed the same procedure for aseptic technique and that techniques were not research based. Breaks in aseptic technique procedures have been implicated in outbreaks of infection (Manning et al. 2001). It is therefore essential that aseptic technique is strictly adhered to when undertaken as well as having a sound theoretical knowledge base regarding aseptic technique and ensuring the procedure is carried out correctly.

Aseptic technique is applied in a number of situations. This includes infection control measures (refer to Chapter 4), the insertion of catheter (refer to Chapter 9) and wound care (refer to Chapter 12). This requires the preparation of the patient, nurse, environment and equipment. Hands need to be washed. Sterile packs, gloves, equipment and solutions are required: a **sterile field** must be created and maintained throughout the procedure. The environment is prepared by drawing the curtains, closing the door, and cleaning the trolley with 70 per cent isopropyl alcohol (before and after use). The patient is prepared by explaining the procedure, gaining their consent and positioning the patient comfortably for the procedure. Antiseptic solution is used to decontaminate the hands. Only sterile supplies (e.g., swabs, fluids) are used. The nurse is prepared by referring to the patient's care plan to ascertain what dressing is to be applied to the wound, following the principles of aseptic technique prior to undertaking the procedure and following evidence based practice and local trust policy.

REFER TO PROCEDURE: ASEPTIC TECHNIQUE

However, a clean technique may be used. A clean technique adopts the same aims as the aseptic technique but uses clean rather than sterile gloves, is less ritualistic and relies on less hand washing between procedures. It still uses sterile equipment and fluids (Gilmour 2000) and the environment is not as crucial as it is for the aseptic technique. The clean technique employs a no-touch technique. Clean, as opposed to sterile, gloves are worn (unless sterile items are handled). The clean technique is used during the following situations:

- when applying dressings to healing wounds by secondary intention
- attending to dressings covering tracheostomy sites
- removing drains or sutures
- ET suction.

Summary

Hand washing is the single most important way of preventing the spread of infection in health care settings. Education and training for all healthcare staff is important in order to prevent the spread of infections and treating those who are affected. Legal and policy obligations must be adhered to and NMC guidelines followed.

LEARNING ACTIVITY 5.2

It is a hot day with temperatures rising to 30 degrees celcius. Fans are switched on and the windows are opened, to allow air to circulate and provide some relief. Prior to undertaking a wound dressing Nurse Jones places her sterile trolley near an open window and fan.
    Is this appropriate? If not, why not?

PROCEDURE: HAND WASHING	
Action	Rationale
Remove rings, bracelets, wristwatches and roll up sleeves	Jewellery inhibits good hand washing; dirt and bacteria can remain beneath jewellery after hand washing and long sleeves can harbour micro-organisms
Cover cuts and abrasions with a waterproof dressing	They can become contaminated with bacteria and cannot be easily cleared. Repeated hand washing can increase injury
Keep nails short and clean. Remove nail varnish and artificial nails	Long false nails can be a source of infection by harbouring dirt and bacteria. Varnish can become cracked resulting in contamination if they fell into wounds. Varnish can also inhibit effective hand washing by potentially harbouring bacteria
Turn taps on with elbows and allow water to flow that doesn't splash and is hand hot	Taps and paper towel dispenser exit most likely areas for contamination and therefore contaminate the hands of the next user Hand-hot water and soap are effective in breaking down dirt and organic matter; ensures surfaces of hands are cleaned and areas are not missed, which can be a source of infection
Wet hands under the running water *before* applying liquid soap/ antimicrobial preparation	Soap applied directly to dry hands may damage the skin Wet hands allow the soap to mix quickly and speed up hand washing

(Cont'd)

Action	Rationale
Apply soap to all of the wet surfaces of the hands and create a lather Wash hands with liquid soap from a dispenser and hand-hot water, if visibly or potentially soiled or contaminated with dirt or organic material	Liquid soap is effective removing dirt, organic material and any transient flora, but has little antimicrobial activity
Rub hands together thoroughly, paying particular attention between the fingers, tips of fingers and thumbs, palms, backs of hands and wrists Rinse soap thoroughly for 10–15 seconds into the hands; 30 seconds preferably	Ensures all surfaces of the hands are cleaned and minimises cross-infection
Rotationally rub wrists palm to palm with fingers interlaced Right palm to back of left hand with fingers interlaced Left palm to back of right hand with fingers interlaced Rotationally rub right thumb in left palm and left thumb with right palm Hold hands upright and rinse under hand-hot water to remove soap Turn taps off with elbows	All surfaces must be thoroughly washed for effective hand washing to have taken place Soap residue can cause skin damage Holding hands upright ensures water splashed from unwashed hands doesn't run on to clean hands Wet hands encourage bacteria growth and may result in sore hands Residue of soap can cause irritation and damage skin resulting in cross-infection So hands are not contaminated with bacteria
Dry hands thoroughly with paper towels and dispose of towels into a foot-operated black bag bin	Damp hands encourage bacteria to multiply and can potentially become sore. Foot-operated bins prevent contamination of the hands Ensure the bins are not overcrowded so the hands are not contaminated Thorough drying minimises micro-organisms and prevents hands becoming sore

PROCEDURE: USING ALCOHOL HAND RUB	
Action	**Rationale**
Hands visibly clean and not soiled or contaminated with dirt or organic material may be cleaned with alcohol hand rub	Hand rubs are a convenient method of cleaning hands but cannot remove organic material or dirt Antimicrobial activity of alcohol able to denature proteins

	A quick convenient method of cleaning hands of gram negative, gram positive, vegetative bacteria, TB and a variety of fungi Has poor activity against bacterial spores and cannot remove dirt or organic material
Rub the alcohol hand rub into all areas of the hands until dry, following manufacturer's instructions	Ensures all areas of the hands are cleaned as alcohol is a rapid acting disinfectant and results in the hands being dry Ensures correct amount of hand rub is used for effective hand cleaning Prevents equipment being contaminated and ensures effective hand cleaning

PROCEDURE: ASEPTIC TECHNIQUE

Action	Rationale
Explain and discuss the procedure with the patient	Ensures understanding and consent gained
Wash hands according to local policy Clean dressing trolley with chlorhexidine or 70 per cent isopropyl alcohol, in accordance with trust policy and ensure the trolley is dry before using	Prevents cross-infection Provides a clean working surface Remove a high proportion of micro-organisms and bacterial spores
Check dressing pack and all other items to be used for the dressing remain intact and within expiry date. If so place all equipment on bottom shelf of dressing trolley. If not intact, discard	Keeps top shelf as a clean working surface Ensures only sterile products are used Areas of contamination are kept to a minimum Reduces risk of infection
Take dressing trolley to the patient disturbing the curtain as little as possible	Minimises airborne contamination
Position patient comfortably for the dressing without exposing them unduly with curtains drawn/door and windows shut	Allow airborne organisms to settle before exposing the sterile field Maintains privacy, dignity and comfort
Wearing a plastic apron, loosen tapes and remove dressing	Reduces risk of cross-infection; eases removal of the dressing and minimises risk of contamination
Clean hands with alcohol hand rub	Reduces the risk of wound infection
Open the dressing package and slide the contents on to the top shelf of the trolley. Create a sterile field using only the corners of the paper	Ensures only sterile products are used Areas of contamination are kept to a minimum Reduces risk of infection

(Cont'd)

Action	Rationale
Tip contents of all other items gently onto the sterile field, e.g., gently pouring solutions into gallipot	
Clean hands again with alcohol hand rub	Hands may be contaminated when handling the packs Reduces risk of cross-infection
Wear gloves touching only the inside wrist end (see procedure regarding sterile gloves)	Reduces the risk of infection Gloves cause less trauma to the patient
Ensure patient is comfortable; adjust the bed to a convenient height; adjust bed clothing and perform the procedure	Avoids stooping; facilitates procedure undertaken; exposes the wound; maintains privacy and dignity
Once procedure is completed dispose of any sharp items into sharps container and all other waste into yellow clinical waste bin; replace bed clothing; ensure patient is comfortable; readjust the bed height and draw back the curtain/open the door/window	Prevents environmental contamination Patient comfort, dignity maintained
Clean hands after disposing of gloves, apron and waste in accordance with trust policy	Reduces the risk of spread of infection
Clean dressing trolley with chlorhexidine/ 70 per cent isopropyl alcohol in accordance with trust policy and paper towels	Reduces the risk of cross-infection
Document care given and condition of wound. Report any changes or abnormalities	Effective communication and ensures care given Evaluates care and wound

PROCEDURE: PUTTING ON STERILE GLOVES

Action	Rationale
Wash hands and dry thoroughly	Prevents cross-infection and contamination of the gloves
Consider the task to be undertaken and choose the correct size of glove Check for integrity and expiry date	Dexterity impaired if incorrect size of glove worn If integrity lost and outside of expiry date gloves no longer sterile
Prepare a large, clean, dry surface for opening the packet containing the gloves by cleaning with 70 per cent isopropyl alcohol/ chlorhexidine, in accordance with local policy Peel open the outer pack from the corners and lay on the surface	To maintain a sterile field

Action	Rationale
Open the inner glove wrapper exposing the cuffed gloves with the palms facing up	Prevents contamination and cross-infection
Pick up the first glove by the cuff touching only the inside portion of the cuff	Prevents contamination and cross-infection
While holding the cuff in one hand, point the glove towards the floor and slip the other hand into the glove	Prevents contamination. If this glove doesn't fit correctly, wait until the second glove is worn and then adjust
Pick up the second glove by sliding the fingers of the gloved hand under the cuff of the second glove. Take care not to contaminate the gloved hand with the ungloved hand while putting on the second glove	Prevents contamination
Put second glove on the ungloved hand by maintaining a steady pull on the cuff. Adjust the gloved fingers until the gloves fit comfortably	To ensure gloves remain sterile. Prevent contamination of the sterile gloves
Discard gloves into the yellow waste bin once use completed. Wash and dry hands thoroughly according to trust policy	

PROCEDURE: GLOVE REMOVAL	
Action	**Rationale**
Grasp one of the gloves near the cuff and pull it part way off. Glove will begin to turn inside out	Keep the first glove partially on before removing the second glove to protect you from touching theoutside surface of either glove with bare hands
Leave the first glove over the fingers, grasp the second glove near the cuff and pull it part way off. Glove will begin to turn inside out	Keep the second glove partially on to protect touching the outside surface of the first glove with bare hands
Pull off the two gloves at the same time touching the inside surface of the gloves	To minimise contamination
Dispose of the gloves into the clinical waste bag and wash hands immediately	Gloves may contain contaminates leaving you at risk of exposure and infection
Avoid letting the gloves snap	To prevent the contaminants splashing into eyes, mouth, face

References

Ayliffe, GAF et al. (2000) *Control of Hospital Infection: A Practical Handbook,* 4th edn. Arnold, London.

Blakemore, MA and Proski, FM (1984) Is Hot Air Hygienic? *Home Economist* 4: 14–15.

Bree-Williams, F and Waterman, H (1996) An Examination of Nurses' Practices When Performing Aseptic Technique for Wound Dressings, *Journal of Advanced Nursing* 2233: 48–54.

Brighton and Sussex University Hospital 2003 http://bsuh.nhs.uk/hospitals/infection-control/infection-control-projects/clean-hands-campaign

Burnett, E et al. (2008) Hand Hygiene: What About Our Patients? *British Journal of Infection Control* 9(1): 19–24.

Burton, RW and Englekirk, PG (2004) *Microbiology for the Health Sciences,* 7th edn. Lippincott Williams and Wilkins, Philadelphia.

Chalmers, C and Straub, M (2006) Standard Principles for Preventing and Controlling Infection, *Nursing Standard* 20(23): 57–65.

Colombo, C et al. (2002) Impact of Teaching Interventions on Nurse Compliance with Hand Disinfection, *Journal of Hospital Infection* 50(1): 69–71.

David, J (1991) Letters, *Wound Management* 1(2): 15.

DH (2001) Standard Principles for Preventing Hospital Acquired Infections, *Journal of Hospital Infection* 47(Suppl): S21–S37.

DH (2005) *Wash Your Hands.* DH, London.

DH (2006) *Health Technical Memorandum 07–01: Safe Management of Healthcare Waste.* DH, London.

Dougherty, L and Lister, S (2008) *Royal Marsden Hospital Manual of Clinical Procedures Student Edition,* 7th edn. Wiley – Blackwell, Oxford.

Driever, R et al. (2001) Surgical Glove Perforation in Cardiac Surgery, *Thoracic Cardiovascular Surgery* 49(6): 328–330.

Gilmour, D (2000) Is the Aseptic Technique Always Necessary? *Journal of Community Nursing* 14(4): 32–35.

Girou, E et al. (2004) Misuse of Gloves: The Foundation for Poor Compliance with Hand Hygiene and Potential for Microbial Transmission? *Journal of Hospital Infection* 57: 162–169.

Gould, D (1994) The Significance of Hand Drying in the Prevention of Infection, *Nursing Times* 90(47): 30–35.

Gould, D (2000) Innovations in Hand Hygiene: Manual from SSL International, *British Journal of Nursing* 9(20): 2175–2180.

Gould, D et al. (2007) The Clean Your Hands Campaign: Critiquing Policy and Evidence Base, *Journal of Hospital Infection* 65(2): 95–101.

Hugonnet, A and Pittet, D (2000) Hand Hygiene – Beliefs or Science? *Clinical Microbiology and Infection* 6(7): 348–354.

ICNA (2007) The Third Prevalence Survey of Hospital Acquired Infection in Acute Hospitals in 2006, ICNA Feb 2007. www.icna.co.uk

Kelsall, NKR et al. (2006) Should Finger Rings be Removed Prior to Scrubbing for Theatre? *Journal of Hospital Infection* 62(4): 450–452.

Kilpatrick, C et al. (2007) 'Germs. Wash Your Hands of Them'. Scotland's Hand Hygiene Campaign. www.scotland.gov.uk

King, D (1998) Determining the Cause of Diarrhoea, *Nursing Times* 98(23): 47–48.

Knight, B et al. (1993) *Hand Drying: A Survey of Efficiency and Hygiene.* Applied Ecology Research Group University of Westminster, London.

Kocent, H et al. (2002) Washing of Gloved Hands in Antiseptic Solution Prior to Central Line Insertion Reduces Contamination, *Anaesthesia and Intensive Care Medicine* 303(3): 338–340.

Lugg, GR and Ahmed, HA (2008) Nurses' Perceptions of Methicillin-Resistant Staphlococcus Aureus: Impacts on Practice, *British Journal of Infection Control* 9(1): 8–14.

Manning, ML et al. (2001) Serratia Marcescens Transmission in a Paediatric Intensive Care Unit: A Multifactorial Occurrence, *American Journal Of Infection Control* 29(2): 115–119.

MHRA (2002) Labelled Single Use Only. One Liners. 19 DH, London.

NAO (2004) Improving Patient Care by Reducing the Risk of Hospital Acquired Infection: A Progress Report. www. nao.org.uk

NHSQIS (2005) Hospital Acquired Infection: Infection Control in NHS Scotland National Overview May 2005. NHSQIS, Edinburgh, Scotland.

NPSA (2004) *Clean Hands Help to Save Lives.* NPSA (Patient Safety Alert 4), London.

NPSA (2004a) *Achieving Our Aims: Evaluating the Results of the Pilot CleanYourHands Campaign.* www.npsa.nhs.uk

NPSA (2007) Homepage www.npsa.nhs.uk/cleanyourhands/the-campaign/background

NICE (2003) *Infection Control Prevention of Healthcare – Associated Infection in Primary and Community Care (No. 1) Standard Principles.* NICE, London.

NMC (2008) *The Code: Standards for Conduct, Performance and Ethics.* NMC, London.

Patrick, DR et al. (1997) Residual Moisture Determines the Level of Touch Contact Associated Bacterial Transfer Following Hand Washing, *Epidemiology Infect* 119(3): 319–325.

Pittet, D et al. (2000) Effectiveness of a Hospital-Wide Programme to Improve Compliance with Hand Hygiene, *Lancet* 356 (9238): 1307–1312.

Pittet, D and Boyce, JM (2001) Hand Hygiene and Patient Care: Pursuing the Semmelweis Legacy, *Lancet Infectious Diseases* April 9–20.

Pittet, D et al. (2004) Hand Hygiene Among Physicians: Performance, Beliefs and Perceptions, *Annals Internal Medicine* 14(4): 1–8.

Porteus, J (2002) Artificial Nails: Very Real Risk, *Canadian Operating Room Nursing* 20(3): 16–17, 20–21.

Randle, J et al. (2006) Hand Hygiene Compliance in Healthcare Workers, *Journal of Hospital Infection* 64(3): 205–209.

Redway, K et al. (1994) *Hand Drying: A Study of Behavioural Types Associated with Different Methods and With Hot Air Dryers.* University of Westminster, London.

RCN (2005) *Good Practice in Infection Prevention and Control Guidance for Nursing Staff.* RCN, London.

RCN (2005a) *Wipe it Out Campaign on MRSA.* www.nric.org.uk

Storr, J and Clayton, S (2004) Hand Hygiene, *Nursing Standard* 18(40): 45–51.

Taylor, JH et al. (2000) A Microbiological Evaluation of Warm Air Hand Driers with Respect to Hand Hygiene and the Washroom Environment, *Journal of Applied Microbiology* 89(6): 910–919.

Ward, S (2000) Hand Washing Facilities in the Clinical Area: A Literature Review, *British Journal of Nursing* 9(2): 82–86.

Whitby, M et al. (2007) Behavioural Consideration for Hand Hygiene Practices: The Basic Building Blocks, *Journal of Hospital Infection* 65(1): 1–8.

Wilson, J (2001) *Infection Control in Clinical Practice,* 2nd edn. Balliere Tindall, Edinburgh.

Whitby, M and McLaws, ML (2004) Handwashing in Healthcare Workers: Accessibility of Sink Location Does Not Improve Compliance, *Hospital Infection* 58: 247–253.

WHO (2005) *Global Patient Safety*. WHO, Geneva.

WHO (2007) *Patient Safety Solutions*. WHO, Geneva.

Xavier, G (1999) Asepsis, *Nursing Standard* 13(36): 49–53.

Yamamoto, Y et al. (2005) Efficiency of Hand Drying for Removing Bacteria from Washed Hands: Comparison of Paper Towel Drying with Warm Air Drying, *Infection Control Hospital Epidemiology* 26(3): 316–320.

6

Vital Signs and Neurological Observations Monitoring

Learning Outcomes

This chapter is designed to help you:

o   understand the principles of monitoring vital signs
o   understand the methods used to observe and record (a) temperature, (b) pulse, (c) respiration, (d) oxygen saturation, (e) blood pressure and (f) neurological observations
o   be aware of complications that may occur when monitoring vital signs
o   understand what action is required when abnormalities occur.

Introduction

The monitoring of vital signs and neurological observations helps to assess an individual's health status and to indicate any changes in that status. The monitoring, recording and interpreting of vital signs and neurological observations enables nurses to make assessments and to plan, implement and evaluate care and treatment. The NMC (2007) identifies that students must be able to 'apply a range of essential nursing skills under the supervision of a registered nurse, to meet individuals' needs, which include taking physiological measurements'.

Temperature Recording

Body temperature represents a balance between heat being generated and heat lost. It is regulated by the **thermoregulatory centre** located in the **hypothalamus** in the brain. Two types of body temperature are recorded: *core* body temperature, which records the temperature in the abdominal cavity and pelvis, where the temperature remains constant; and *surface* temperature, which records the temperature of the skin, **subcutaneous tissue** and fat, where the temperature fluctuates due to the environment.

The ability of the body to maintain its temperature is achieved by mechanisms that conserve heat and others that promote heat loss. These are, respectively, **vasoconstriction** (piloerection, shivering, heat conservation) and **vasodilation** (increased sweating, increased rate and depth of respiration, reduced metabolism to promote heat loss). Recording body temperature serves several functions. It establishes a patient's baseline temperature; indicates any changes, e.g., basal metabolic conditions, for example in the case of post-operative care, critically ill patients, immunosuppressed patients, patients with an infection, pyrexial patients, those receiving a blood transfusion; and indicates fluctuations such as **hypothermia** and **hyperthermia** (**pyrexia**) and patients' responses to **antipyretics** and antibiotics.

Body temperature is recorded in degrees celcius. It should range between 36–37.5 degrees celcius, to maintain metabolic activity (as it needs to be relatively constant for cellular metabolism), but this varies according to the site used. Body temperature also responds to the environmental temperature and fluctuates according to time of day due to circadian rhythms. Temperature will tend to be lower at six o'clock in the morning and higher at six o'clock in the evening (Marieb and Hoehn 2007).

Because of these variations, consistency in monitoring and recording is required. Numerous other factors affect the temperature (some of which are identified in Box 6.1).

Box 6.1   Factors Affecting Temperature

Ovulation (progesterone secretion and basal metabolic rate influences increases temperature)
Consuming hot/cold drinks
Smoking
Environment
Age (reduced thermoregulatory efficiency, inactivity, loss of subcutaneous fat in the elderly, immature control system in children until puberty leaves them vulnerable to temperature fluctuations)
Exercise (increases body temperature)
Stress (sympathetic nervous system stimulates increasing **epinephrine** and **norepinephrine**)

(Brooker and Waugh 2007, Dougherty and Lister 2008)

Temperature may be recorded orally, axillary, rectally or **auditory** using a digital analogue probe or **tympanic** device. When recording temperature orally, the thermometer is placed in the **sublingual** pocket under the tongue and towards the back of the mouth. For tympanic recordings, a tympanic device is used. This must be fitted with a protective cover before it is inserted into the ear. Both sites allow ease of access for temperature recording. Rectal temperature recordings are accurate but rarely used and not recommended for patients with a myocardial infarction (as vagal stimulation causes myocardial damage), or those who have undergone rectal surgery, or are suffering from diarrhoea or haemorrhoids (Trim 2005).

The axilla is the preferred site for patients who have undergone oral surgery, had their jaws wired, or are unable to mouth or nose breathe, and also for confused individuals and newborns. However, it is a less reliable and less accurate site than others (Evans et al. 1994) as it is not close to major vessels (Woollens 1996). Oral and axillary sites are exposed to the cooling effects of ambient temperature, while rectal temperature is lower due to the heat generated from metabolic activity of micro-organisms in the rectum.

LEARNING ACTIVITY 6.1

Identify the reasons for recording temperatures at the following sites and, in each case, the advantages and disadvantages:

- Oral
- Tympanic
- Axilla
- Rectum

Hypothermia is defined as a core body temperature below 35 degrees celcius and can cause the metabolic rate to decrease (Trim 2005). It can be described as mild, moderate or severe hypothermia (Brooker and Waugh 2007). Mild hypothermia is where the temperature ranges between 32 and 35 degrees celcius while moderate hypothermia is where the temperature ranges between 28 and 32 degrees celcius. Severe hypothermia is where the body's temperature is below 28 degrees celcius (Cuddy 2004). This occurs when the body loses more heat and is subsequently unable to maintain homeostasis (Ncho 2005).

Hypothermia frequently escapes detection: the symptoms are non-specific and oral thermometers fail to record within an appropriate range (Marini and Wheeler 2006). The elderly are at particular risk for a number of reasons. These include:

- environmental exposure
- medication (which alters perception of the cold and can lead to increased heat loss through vasodilatation or heat inhibition generation)
- metabolic conditions (for example, hypoglycaemia, adrenal insufficiency and in post-operative situations when anaesthetic drugs are administered, dampening vasoconstrictor response) (Marini and Wheeler 2006).

Hyperthermia or pyrexia occurs when there is a significant rise in body temperature (Marieb and Hoehn 2007). This may be caused either by infection or other causes, such as consumption of hot drinks or a reaction to a transfusion or drug. Mild or low grade pyrexia ranges between 37 and 38 degrees celcius. Temperature in this range may indicate an inflammatory response to a mild infection, allergy or body tissue disturbance.

Moderate or high grade hyperthermia is associated with temperatures in the range between 38 to 40 degrees celcius. Such temperatures may be caused by a wound, respiratory or urinary tract infection. Hyperpyrexia occurs when temperatures exceed 40 degrees celcius. Typical causes include bacteraemia, damage of the hypothalamus or a high environmental temperature (Dougherty and Lister 2008).

It is vitally important to monitor body temperature carefully: an inaccurate recording can result if an inappropriate site is used, or if external factors are not considered when recording a temperature.

REFER TO PROCEDURE: TAKING A TEMPERATURE VIA TYMPANIC ROUTE

Pulse Recording

The pulse is the rhythmic expansion and relaxation of the elastic arteries caused by the ejection of blood from the left ventricle when it contracts. It is the rhythmic pulsation of the blood and represents a **heart rate** when any artery is palpated close to the body surface. When taking the pulse, one needs to note the rate, rhythm and strength to ascertain the patient's state of health.

The pulse is dependent upon the degree of activity and the **autonomic nervous system** (ANS) whereby stimulation of the sympathetic nervous system and release of **adrenaline** increases the heart rate. Stimulation of the **parasympathetic nervous system** has the opposite effect by reducing the heart rate. This is influenced by cardiac output, stroke volume and heart rate. It is also influenced by neural, chemical and physical factors induced by homeostatic mechanisms, e.g., sympathetic and parasympathetic nervous systems, hormones, electrolytes, stress and exercise (Marieb and Hoehn 2007, Thibodeau and Patton 2007).

Cardiac output refers to the amount of blood pumped out by each ventricle. It is measured over a period of one minute. Stroke volume is the amount of blood pumped out by the ventricle with each contraction. This can be expressed as follows:

$$cardiac\ output = heart\ rate \times stroke\ volume$$

(Marieb and Hoehn 2007)

Thus if the blood volume drops, stroke volume declines and cardiac output is maintained by increasing the heart rate.

An increase in the pulse rate is referred to as **tachycardia** and is reflected by an abnormally fast heart rate (greater than 100 beats per minute). It may be caused by **hypovolaemia**, increased pain, pyrexia, shock, stress, dehydration, medication, heart disease, infection or exercise. **Bradycardia** (below 60 beats per minute) is a slow heart rate and may be induced by sleep, hypothermia, drugs, myocardial infarction or intracranial pressure. **Fibrillation** is the rapid and irregular contraction of the heart (e.g., atrial fibrillation, ventricular fibrillation). A weak pulse may indicate decreased cardiac function (McCance and Huether 2006).

The pulse can be recorded at the following sites – temporal (NB useful for children), carotid, brachial, radial, femoral, popliteal (i.e. behind the knee – this is uncommonly used), and pedal pulse. It is achieved by pressing on the artery against a firm tissue and by counting the number of beats during one minute. It is taken to assess cardiovascular function, establish a normal heart rate, rhythm, check the regularity and quality of the pulse rate (**arrhythmia**), monitor response to treatment or surgery, blood transfusion, and establish cardiovascular status and illness. Due to their higher metabolic rate, children have a higher pulse rate compared to adults (as identified in Table 6.1).

Table 6.1   *Normal resting heart rates for adults and children*

Age	Beats per Minute
1 week–3 months	100–160
3 months–2 years	80–150
2–10 years	70–110
10 years–adult	55–90

(Weber and Kelly 2003)

Pulse records should be used in conjunction with the observations of other vital signs, e.g., blood pressure. Raised pulse and reduced blood pressure may indicate haemorrhaging.

A fast, weak, thready pulse may indicate dehydration, hypovolaemia or heart failure. A strong, bounding, fast pulse may indicate pyrexia, anxiety or haemorrhaging. An irregular pulse may indicate heart disease.

It is important to be aware of factors that may affect the patient's pulse, such as pain, fear, anger, pregnancy, alcohol, infection, medication (digoxin reduces heart rate, salbutamol increases pulse rate), exercise (an athlete has a greater cardiac size, strength, efficiency compared to an inactive individual), pyrexia and stress (sympathetic nervous stimulation increases the pulse).

LEARNING ACTIVITY 6.2

- For each of the sites that may be used for recording a pulse, identify the reasons for selecting that site.
- Identify which site is used for (i) an adult, (ii) child, (iii) a person with a mental health problem, and (iv) person with a learning disability.

In children under the age of six years the most accurate way of recording a pulse is to use the apical (apex) site. To record the apical (apex) pulse, the correct use and placing of a stethoscope in children is dependent upon the age of the child: for those under seven years of age, the stethoscope should be placed at the fourth intercostal space and slightly lateral to the left midclavicular line: for those over seven years of age, the fifth intercostal space on the left midclavicular line should be the site (Wong et al. 2001). Effective use of the stethoscope can be difficult if the child is uncooperative. It may be possible to gain the child's cooperation by providing explanations, involving the family, or demonstrating on toys.

REFER TO PROCEDURE: TAKING A PULSE

Respiratory Rate Recording

Respiration is the process of exchanging air between the lungs and the external environment. This involves the intake of oxygen and expulsion of carbon dioxide through the diffusion of

Table 6.2   *Respiratory rates in adults and children*

Age	Respiratory Rate per Minute
Newborn–6 months	30–50
6 months–2 years	20–30
3–10 years	20–28
10–18 years	12–20
Adults	15–20

(Weber and Kelley 2003)

gases. Respiration is controlled through voluntary and involuntary mechanisms regulated by the respiratory centre in the **medulla oblongata, pons** in the brain and **chemoreceptors** located in the medulla, carotid and aortic bodies. These centres and receptors respond to changes in oxygen and carbon dioxide concentrations in arterial blood.

One respiration is counted as one complete inspiration and expiration. Respiratory rate varies with age as noted in Table 6.2. During inspiration the **diaphragm** contracts, the ribs move upwards and outwards, the sternum moves outward, the thorax enlarges and the lungs expand. During expiration the diaphragm relaxes, ribs move down and inwards, the sternum moves inward, the thorax size decreases and the lungs are compressed. During this whole process oxygen enters the lungs and then the alveoli (inspiration) while carbon dioxide is expired (expiration).

At rest the respiratory rate should be regular, effortless and quiet. The rate, depth, pattern, rhythm, and sound may all change as a result of exercise, breathing difficulties, pain, pyrexia, drugs, sleep or alcohol.

REFER TO PROCEDURE: RECORDING RESPIRATORY RATE

The primary purpose of respiratory assessment is to determine the adequacy of gaseous exchange (i.e., the exchange of oxygen and carbon dioxide). Other purposes include: identifying the baseline rate for future comparisons; monitoring changes in oxygenation or respiration; evaluating the response to medication or treatment that affects the respiratory system (Tortora and Derrickson 2008); helping diagnosis; and monitoring fluctuations in a patient's condition.

When undertaking a respiratory assessment the patient should, if possible, be placed in an upright position. This assists lung expansion and access to the thorax. Clothing should be loosened to assist visibility and **auscultation**. Questions asked should be closed ones: this will minimise any distress in the breathless patient. One needs to assess the rate, rhythm, quality and effort taken. Assess how hard the patient is breathing, whether each side is moving equally and what muscles are being used. Listen for noises such as wheezing or gasping. Note that the flaring of nostrils in children indicates respiratory distress (children are nose breathers).

Respiratory function can be affected by pregnancy (due to fluid retention, increased oestrogen levels causing oedema, increased progesterone levels), obesity (impeding lung expansion), circulatory problems (oedema and anaemia impeding lung expansion), environmental influences (e.g., coldness), trauma and pathophysiological problems (e.g., bowel obstruction, ascites). The respiratory rhythm may also be altered as a result of an impaired respiratory centre in the brain.

This may occur, for example, with neurological patients where there is damage or a poor blood supply to the brain stem, resulting in an irregular rhythm and rate (Cheyne–Stoke breathing). A reduction in respirations, respiratory rate and its depth occurs prior to cardiopulmonary arrest. Lips, nail bed, mucous membrane, tips of nose and ear lobes should be closely monitored for cyanosis (Woodrow 2005) if deprived of oxygen, indicating a deterioration in the patient's condition.

Hypoventilation refers to shallow slow breathing, while **hyperventilation** refers to fast and deep breathing. Noisy breathing includes wheezing due to airway constriction on expiration with bronchitis or asthma, while **stridor** is due to an obstruction during inspiration. Mouth breathing, pursing of lips on expiration, use of abdominal muscles or flaring of nostrils requires monitoring because they may indicate underlying potential problems (Field 2000).

Babies have a less regular respiratory rhythm (possibly due to an incomplete development of the normal respiratory control system). Children's lungs are not yet fully developed until the age of three years. The chest wall is softer and more compliant and their airways are narrower: this increases the risk of an obstruction occurring due to inflammation or secretions (Chandler 2001).

To monitor and record the respiratory rate place the baby in a calm and relaxed atmosphere and lightly place the hand on the abdomen in order to count the breaths. If this is not possible, observe the baby while it is playing or interacting with a parent. For babies under 12 months of age, a stethoscope is used to listen for air movement into the lungs. Babies under three months are obligatory nose breathers and therefore are at greater risk of respiratory distress secondary to secretions obstructing the nasal passages (Helms 2000). Always monitor children and babies who flare their nostrils, as it can indicate acute respiratory distress (Field 2000). Any irregularities should be noted and reported immediately to the person in charge and medical team as the condition will dictate the frequency of recording. Children also have higher metabolic rates and accompanying oxygen demand due to immature muscle development. As a result, children compensate well for mild breathing difficulties. However, this may result in muscle fatigue and sudden respiratory failure.

Oxygen Saturations

Oxygen saturation is a measure of the percentage of haemoglobin molecules (Dougherty and Lister 2008) saturated by oxygen. It provides a useful indicator of the amount of oxygen in the peripheries. A pulse oximeter is used to detect the amount of red and infrared light passed through the capillary bed when a probe is placed on the finger or toe. It requires a pulsating blood flow for an accurate recording. Finger tips and ear lobes are generally used with specifically designed probes for oxygen saturations, although the bridge of the nose may sometimes be used (Higgins 2005).

This makes pulse oximetry a non–invasive and simple means of monitoring the percentage of haemoglobin saturated with oxygen in the peripheral blood vessels. It also helps to assess the severity of a patient's condition, i.e., monitoring and evaluating the effectiveness of oxygen therapy, respiratory illness (e.g., asthma), monitoring oxygen status, sedation or anaesthesia.

Readings may be affected by the use of nail varnish (this reduces the translucency of the fingertip, thereby affecting the reading), dirt, foreign objects, anaemia, hypotension, poor circulation, cardiac arrhythmias, rigors or shivering (Woodrow 1999), vasonconstriction, shock (Howell 2002) and poor positioning of the probe. Oximeters do not provide information regarding levels of carbon dioxide or acid–base levels and therefore have limitations when assessing patients progressing into respiratory failure (due to carbon dioxide retention), haemoglobin concentration, or oxygen delivered to the tissues or respiratory function. They thus provide only limited information about a patient's condition. They may, however, be useful when used in conjunction with other assessment tools (Higgins 2005).

REFER TO PROCEDURE: PULSE OXIMETRY

Blood Pressure Monitoring

Blood pressure (BP) is the force of blood exerted on the wall of an artery. It is maintained by a combination of neural, chemical and renal control measures. BP is dependent upon cardiac output (amount of blood ejected by the heart every minute), blood volume, peripheral resistance (the force exerted against the blood vessel wall as blood flows through the blood vessel) and elasticity of the arterioles (which contribute to the resistance) (Thibodeau and Patton 2007, Tortora and Derrickson 2008). It is recorded as two measurements (systolic and diastolic pressure) and is expressed in millimetres of mercury (mmHg).

Blood pressure is measured after the patient has sat at rest in a quiet room for 5–15 minutes. The cuff should be of an appropriate size. Blood pressure cuff sizes for mercury sphygmomanometer, semiautomatic and ambulatory monitors are indicated in Table 6.3.

Systolic blood pressure is caused by the contraction of ventricles and peak pressure of blood in the arteries. **Diastolic blood pressure** occurs when the ventricles relax and there is the minimum pressure of blood against the blood vessel wall, following closure of the aortic valve (Dougherty and Lister 2006). Stroke volume increases with age, while the heart rate falls. Children have a comparatively smaller stroke volume and a higher output than adults as they do not possess a cardiac reserve of an adult. Thus when children are faced with severe blood or fluid loss, they become critically ill quickly.

Blood pressure monitoring can be recorded, either by non-invasive or invasive methods, to: ascertain the baseline blood pressure of the patient; assess response to treatment or illness; aid diagnosis of disease; monitor fluctuations; assess the cardiovascular system during and after

Table 6.3   *Blood pressure cuff sizes*

Indication	Bladder Width × Length	Arm Circumference
Small adult/child	12 × 18	< 23
Standard adult	12 × 26	< 33
Large adult	12 × 40	< 50
Adult thigh cuff	20 × 42	< 53

www.attract.wales.nhs.uk

disease, surgery or trauma; and assess the efficacy of antihypertensive medication and screening, e.g., hypertension, kidney disease. The frequency of recording blood pressure is dependent upon the patient's condition: critically-ill patients have their blood pressure recorded more frequently compared to an active, fit athlete.

The British Hypertension Society (2004) provides the following guidelines for measuring blood pressure.

Box 6.2 Measuring Blood Pressure

- Use a device with validated accuracy that is properly maintained and calibrated.
- Patient should be seated with their arm at the same level as the heart. Bladder size should be adjusted for the arm circumference, the cuff deflated at 2 mmls and blood pressure measured to the nearest 2 mmHg. Diastolic pressure is recorded when the sounds disappear.
- Two measurements should be taken (1–2 minutes apart) to determine blood pressure thresholds.

(British Hypertension Society 2004)

Box 6.3 How to Record Blood Pressure

- Sit the patient at rest for five minutes in a calm, quiet environment.
- Support the arm at the level of the heart.
- The cuff size should fit the arm (covering more than 80 per cent of the circumference of the arm). The lower edge of the cuff is placed two centimetres below the antecubital fossa and the stethoscope bell is placed over the brachial artery.
- An appropriately maintained device should be used.
- Rapid inflation of the cuff.
- Estimate the systolic blood pressure by **palpation.**
- Reinflate the cuff and slowly deflate 2–3 mmHg per second.
- The first appearance of regular sounds is the systolic blood pressure (unless the patient is in atrial fibrillation).
- Disappearance of the sounds is the diastolic blood pressure (unless patient pregnant).
- Take two separate measurements.
- Record the measurement.
- Explain the result.

(British Hypertension Society 2004)

The blood pressure of newborns, infants and children is measured and recorded less frequently than for adults. With children under the age of one year, the thigh is used to record blood pressure. With babies, blood pressure is recorded when they are asleep or resting.

Mercury sphygmomanometers are reliable: they remain the gold standard for measuring blood pressure, provided they are properly maintained and used according to strict criteria (refer to British Hypertension Society 2004 recommendations). Aneroid devices are widely used, but the monitors are notoriously difficult to maintain in an accurate state over time and are not recommended for routine use. Ambulatory blood pressure monitoring (ABPM) provides more information than home or clinic measurements as it provides a 24–hour profile of blood pressures recorded. However, they are only validated when a well maintained machine with an appropriate cuff size is used (O'Brien et al. 2003).

For home or self-monitored blood pressure measurement, validated, well maintained machines with appropriate cuff sizes should be used (British Hypertension Society 2004). There are advantages to such monitoring, including the availability of multiple recordings throughout the day and avoidance of the 'white coat effect'. The disadvantages include reporting bias and the risk of unsupervised alteration of medication.

According to the British Hypertension Society, optimal blood pressure is 120/80 mmHg, with normal blood pressure defined as systolic blood pressure no greater than 130 mmHg and diastolic blood pressure no greater than 85 mmHg (Williams et al. 2004). High-to-normal systolic blood pressure is 130–139 mmHg, with diastolic blood pressure 85–89 mmHg (EHS 2003, WHO 1999). Any recording should not be based on one reading alone but a number of consecutive readings, to provide consistency and ensure accuracy.

Hypertension can be an indication of cardiovascular disease, trauma or a side effect of medication, raised intracranial pressure, stress or pain. Approximately 30 per cent of people over 50 years of age are hypertensive (Marieb and Hoehn 2007). **Hypotension** is where the systolic blood pressure is below 100 mmHg and reflects changes such as shock and haemorrhaging. The following factors all affect blood pressure: sodium and water retention, hormones (adrenaline, anti-diuretic hormone, rennin), stress, obesity (increases risk of hypertension), increased blood volume, vasoconstriction, exercise (increases the cardiac output and as a result blood pressure), medication, age (stimulating the sympathetic nervous system increasing cardiac output and vaso-constricting the arterioles thereby altering blood pressure, inhibited vasomotor centre and vasodilatation reducing blood pressure), haemorrhaging, dehydration and alcohol.

REFER TO PROCEDURE: BLOOD PRESSURE MONITORING

Neurological Observations

Neurological observation involves the examination of a patient's nervous system to assess response to various stimuli. It is a way of obtaining objective data on the functioning of the nervous system (Hickey 2003) and evaluating the integrity of an individual's nervous system. Such observation helps to: identify changes occurring in the brain; determine whether urgent intervention is required or what progress a patient is making; diagnose a neurological disease; and monitor the effects and treatment of a neurological disease (Carlson 2002, Kaye 2005). Accurate observation and prompt action can improve the eventual outcome in terms of patient survival and also minimise the degree of residual neurological deficit (Waterhouse 2005).

Areas of Observation

Neurological observations employ a range of measurements and criteria in order to establish changes occurring within the skull. They will indicate whether an individual's neurological status is improving, deteriorating or remaining stable (Shah 1999, Waterhouse 2005). Neurological observation uses a chart which incorporates the Glasgow Coma Score (GCS), allowing key areas to be assessed and recorded.

The chart allows for a quick and repeated evaluation of neurological status (Auken and Crawford 1998, Shah 1999, Waterhouse 2005, Dawson and Shah 2006, Dawes et al. 2007). Three types of response are independently assessed and recorded on a chart – best motor response, best verbal response and eye opening. A score of 15 indicates a normally functioning cerebrum. The lowest score that can be achieved is three, indicating total unresponsiveness (Waterhouse 2005). A deterioration overall is clinically significant and must be reported and acted upon immediately.

Levels of Consciousness

Hickey (2002) defines consciousness as 'a general awareness of oneself and the environment' and may result from an attack on the structures that control consciousness in the brain, lack of food, or toxic effects of endogenous or exogenous substances (drugs) on anatomical structures of the brain. For instance, a direct attack on the head may result in unconsciousness. The level of consciousness is recorded on a Glasgow Coma Score (GCS).

The GCS is a tool for detecting and monitoring changes in a patient's neurological condition. It is designed to grade the severity of impaired consciousness in patients with traumatic head injury or intracranial pressure. It provides an objective, reliable and easy to use measure of consciousness level.

However, it is important to ensure that the baseline record is accurate. Without an accurate baseline score, any future observation and GCS will not provide a reliable indication of changes in the patient's neurological condition or responses to treatment to the underlying condition (Waterhouse 2005).

Assessment of the level of consciousness needs to take into account all of the following: eye opening; verbal and motor response; papillary activity (including size, shape, equality, reaction to light – whether deviated upwards or downwards); and motor function assessment and evaluation for muscle strength, tone, coordination, reflexes and abnormal movements. Assessment of sensory functions involves assessment of central and peripheral vision, hearing and the patient's ability to understand verbal communication and to respond to superficial sensations (light, touch, pain) and deep sensations (muscle and joint pain).

LEARNING ACTIVITY 6.3

Locate the neurological chart in your clinical area.

- Familiarise yourself with the chart.
- Ensure you are clear how the chart should be completed.

Assessing Pupil Size and Reaction

Spontaneously reacting pupils demonstrate that the **reticular-activating system** (RAS) has been stimulated and the patient is aware of their environment. Patients in a persistent vegetative state, however, will open their eyes as a direct reflex action generated by the RAS (Waterhouse 2005). Pupil size should be measured when the pupil is at rest and not when the light is shone into the eye, as importance is placed upon the pupil dilating again after constriction once the light source has been removed (not just on the constriction itself). Dilation demonstrates a higher level of functioning in that the brain has recognised the light has gone and it is satisfactory to dilate again.

Changes in pupil size along with changes in consciousness level may indicate changes in intracranial pressure. Sluggish or suddenly dilated unequal pupils indicate oedema or a haematoma is worsening and the oculomotor cranial nerve is being compressed. Expanding lesions can also affect pupil size by placing pressure on the third cranial nerve. Thus eye opening does not always indicate that neurological function is intact as patients in a persistent vegetative state will open their eyes as a direct reflex act, generated by the RAS (Waterhouse 2005). Those in a long-term coma may open their eyes widely but still be unaware of their surroundings, so accurate assessment is essential.

The eyes should open spontaneously to verbal commands: this indicates the functioning of the arousal mechanisms in the brain stem. Eye opening is a response to a painful stimulus, indicating that neuronal pathways within the RAS are connected to the sensory and motor pathway and are still functioning to some effect. If the patient's eyes are still closed, arousal and opening can be assessed by the degree of stimulation required. For instance, verbal stimulation should produce a response. If this fails to occur, a pain stimulus could be applied to the trapezius muscle (Dawson and Shah 2006) while verbal responses provide information regarding the patient's response to speech, comprehension and functioning areas of the cognitive centres in the brain, and reflects their ability to respond to questions posed (Waterhouse 2005, Dawson and Shah 2006).

Assessing Limb Power in All Limbs (Motor and Sensory Function)

Verbal commands are used to assess movement of the limbs and the degree of dysfunction. Each limb should be assessed separately by asking the patient to hold their arms out and noting for signs of weakness, or resistance, when the limb is pushed down or away. If abnormal responses to touch occur it may be due to the loss of sensation (anaesthetic), greater than normal sensation (**hyperaesthesia**), or less than normal sensation (**hypoaesthesia**). These should be reported and documented.

Asking the patient if they know where they are helps to assess their awareness of their surroundings and to show whether they are orientated or confused. The question may be met with inappropriate or incomprehensible responses, or no response at all. A lack of a verbal response may indicate a lack of brain stem activity, age-related communication difficulty (so such a test may not be used for those under the age of five), learning difficulty or damage in the Broca's speech centre or Wernicke's speech centre (Dawson and Shah 2006), language barriers (if English is not the first language spoken) or if a pre-existing problem (for example, a stroke) exists.

Testing motor responses is seen as the most reliable way of assessing consciousness as it tests the patient's response to a painful stimuli (such as a trapezius pinch): this tests the response of the brain that identifies sensory input and translates this into a motor response. The upper limbs should be tested using simple commands such as asking the patient to obey commands, e.g., squeezing the examiner's hands and the best motor response recorded, i.e., power in the hands and the patient's ability to release the grip. This is because some patients with cerebral dysfunction may show an involuntary grasp reflex, where stimulation of the palm causes them to grasp (Auken and Crawford 1998). Responses in the lower limbs reflect spinal function (Auken and Crawford 1998 in Dougherty and Lister 2008).

When assessing motor responses, record the response from the best arm using central painful stimulus, as it is the brain that is being assessed *not* the spinal response. Spinal reflexes may cause the limb to flex briskly and even occur in patients certified as brainstem dead (Stewart 1996), while some patients may mimic what they have seen or been told to do. This would result in errors when interpreting the response. Caution is required because patients with cerebral dysfunction may show an involuntary grasp reflex if the palm of their hand is stimulated, thereby causing a gripping action. An abnormal extension reflects disturbance of the midbrain or pons, while an abnormal flexion indicates malfunction in the brain stem (Palmer and Knight 2006).

As the level of consciousness is the most sensitive indicator of neurological deterioration, any neurological changes should be readily identifiable, unless the patient is receiving a sedative or anaesthetic. Observation of the neurological status in children is a complex skill requiring knowledge of child development. Observation of a child should be performed by the same nurse on each occasion so that any subtle changes are not missed (Grant et al. 1990). Using the GCS to assess a child's level of consciousness is unreliable because developmental milestones may not have been reached and language skills may not have developed. Also, GCS assessment is problematic with children with verbal communication difficulties or a learning disability or where English is not their first language. The GCS assessment should be performed only as part of a much more comprehensive neurological observation and not carried out by students. Instead, focus upon observing the patient for eye opening (arousal), verbal and motor responses.

REFER TO PROCEDURE: NEUROLOGICAL OBSERVATION

Measuring and Recording Vital Signs

A reduction in pulse, raised blood pressure and irregular respiratory rate, along with **Cushing's triad** or **reflex**, are indications of rising intracranial pressure. Here the patient is in danger of 'coning' (**cerebral herniation**). Combined with altered consciousness level or vomiting, this requires immediate and medical intervention as it can lead to death.

Hypertension occurs with an increase in systolic blood pressure combined with widening pulse pressure. This causes systemic vasoconstriction and an increase in blood pressure. Bradycardia allows the systole to pump more blood at a higher pressure, forcing blood into the brain during peak arterial systolic blood pressure. An irregular respiratory rate is due to impaired respiratory centre in the pons and medulla.

Pyrexia may occur due to infection or a severe head injury causing damage to the temperature-regulating centre in the hypothalamus. As the temperature increases, cerebral cell metabolism results in excess carbon dioxide and vasodilation of the cerebral blood vessels, compounding any existing swelling.

Summary

Vital signs and neurological observations can help to ensure that care is tailored to the individual needs of the patient and assessment. Monitoring vital signs and neurological observations are crucial in patient care in order to detect ill health or evaluate patient progress. They provide information regarding general health and cardiovascular and neurological status, which will dictate the frequency of the observation required. Observations should be recorded and considered in conjunction with each other, not in isolation. It is important to relate observations to the baseline measurements for the patient, not rely on textbook values. Any abnormality must be reported for prompt and immediate intervention.

Scenarios

All adapted from Baille (2001: 33–4).

Consider the following questions in relation to the scenarios.

- How would you approach each patient in order to take their vital signs/neurological observations?
- Using your communication skills to date and what you have learnt in Chapter 3, how would you communicate with each patient?

Adult

Roy Atkinson, a 70 year old gentleman, is taken to a medical unit by ambulance following a suspected cerebro vascular accident (CVA). He was found on the floor at home. Some of Roy's family, including his 69 year old wife and daughter in her 30s are with him. They seem very anxious about him.

Child

Kevin O'Riordan is a 14 year old boy who has undergone an operation to remove a perforated appendix, which led to peritonitis (an inflammation and infection of the lining of the abdominal cavity). Kevin has a surgical wound on his abdomen, is receiving intravenous fluids and is nil by mouth. He seems quiet and uncommunicative. Kevin has two younger sisters and his parents spend part of every day with him in hospital.

Mental Health

Vera Wilson, an 80 year old lady, has been admitted again to a ward for the elderly and mentally infirm with a marked deterioration in her mental state. Her mood is low and she appears confused, disorientated, agitated and restless. She also seems very frightened.

Learning Disabilities

Clara Wright is a 43 year old lady with a learning disability who lives in a small staffed unit. She has epilepsy and this morning, had a prolonged seizure for which a muscle relaxant (diazepam) was given. She is now very drowsy, unresponsive and you have been told that her respiration and blood pressure need to be monitored carefully.

Critical Reflection

Mr Kellor, a 72 year old man, is admitted via the Emergency Department with an acute onset of shortness of breath, chest pain and anxiety. The initial assessment shows cyanosis of the lips and nail beds, an oxygen saturation rate of 83 per cent and respiratory rate of 22.

- From your experience and studies to date what would you do here?
- To whom would you report the outcome of your assessment?

Mrs James, a 42 year old lady is recovering from a total abdominal hysterectomy. The nurse notes during her assessment on the first post-operative day that Mrs James is disorientated, hypotensive and tachycardic.

- From your experiences and studies to date what would you do here?
- To whom would you report your findings, if anyone?

From your studies and practice to date test yourself on the following questions:

1 What factors could affect a person's ability to respond verbally?
2 What difficulties would there be when assessing children's motor response?
3 What factors could affect the assessment of an individual?
4 What are the common causes of hypertension?
5 What could affect the accuracy of blood pressure recording?
6 Which possible factors may affect pulse rates?
7 What factors affect the respiratory rate?
8 What might affect a patient's temperature?
9 How would you record a child's temperature?
10 What are the causes of pyrexia?
11 What are the causes of hypothermia?
12 Shivering is activated by which organ when the shell temperature falls below 35 degrees celcius?
13 The body can only function within a narrow temperature range. What is this range?

PROCEDURE: TAKING A TEMPERATURE VIA TYMPANIC ROUTE

Action	Rationale
Explain and discuss the procedure and obtain consent	Ensure patient understanding and any consent obtained is informed and valid
Wash and dry hands thoroughly	Minimises risk of cross-infection and contamination
Using tympanic thermometer remove thermometer from base unit and ensure lens clean. Use dry wipe to clean	Alcohol-based wipes produce false results, i.e., a low temperature
Place disposable probe cover over probe tip	Probe cover protects the tip and functioning of instrument
Gently place probe tip into ear canal to seal opening and snug fit	Prevents air at ear opening entering the ear and producing a low temperature
Press SCAN button Remove from ear once recording taken	Commences scanning Ensures reading undertaken and recorded
Read temperature and document	Ensures reading recorded
Press RELEASE/EJECT button to discard probe cover and replace thermometer into base unit	To charge battery

PROCEDURE: TAKING A PULSE

Action	Rationale
Explain and discuss with the patient the procedure and obtain consent. Ask if they have exercised or been active in the last 15 minutes	Ensures patient understanding and consent obtained is informed and valid. Activity increases the heart rate and consequently increases the pulse rate
Ensure patient is comfortable and ensure recording is under same conditions as previous recordings	Ensures continuity and consistency in the recordings
Place three fingers along appropriate artery, i.e., radial artery and press gently not using the index finger	Fingertips are sensitive to touch but don't use thumb or index finger to avoid recording own pulse
Count for 60 seconds if irregular; if regular count for 30 seconds and double. Note the patient skin colour for pallor, cyanosis. Document results	Sufficient time to detect any irregularities or other defects. Observing for anaemia, cyanosis, oxygen circulating around the body. To ensure reading recorded
For children under 2 years of age avoid this approach. Use a stethoscope and listen to apical heart beat	Inaccurate results obtained. Obtains accurate results

PROCEDURE: RECORDING RESPIRATORY RATE

Action	Rationale
Ensure patient is relaxed prior to the procedure and observe chest rise and fall for 60 seconds covertly	Ensures patient breathing naturally To establish regular rate and rhythm
Observe for rate, rhythm and depth, respiratory effort, i.e., nasal flaring, pursed lips, use of accessory muscles	Indicates patient making extra effort when breathing and may indicate changes in respiratory status
Listen for cough or wheezing; cyanosis; symmetry in chest movement; difficulty in breathing/pain	Dry cough indicates viral infection, bronchial cancer Moist cough indicates bronchitis, asthma, bacterial infection Wheezing indicates bronchospasm
Document and report any abnormalities	Early identification of any underlying medical problem

PROCEDURE: BLOOD PRESSURE MONITORING

Action	Rationale
Explain and discuss the procedure with the patient Obtain consent	Ensures patient understanding and consent obtained is informed and valid
Allow patient to rest before recording	Ensures accurate recording obtained Seated position achieves best results
Support upper arm, positioned at heart level and palm upwards Remove any tight or restrictive clothing	Obtains accurate reading Dangling arm at hip level equates to 11–12 mmHg higher reading thereby giving a false reading Obtains an accurate recording
Cover 80 per cent of the upper arm circumference with blood pressure cuff, 2–3 cms above the brachial artery Cuff should fit snugly around the arm ensuring centre of the cuff covers brachial artery and is at level of heart	Obtains an accurate recording Obtains an accurate recording
Position sphygmomanometer close to the patient, at eye level and on a firm surface	Obtains an accurate recording Ensures equipment not caught on anything loose
Inflate cuff until artery can no longer be felt/heard; usually 30 mmHg above estimated systolic pressure	Prevents blood flow through artery

(Cont'd)

Action	Rationale
Place diaphragm of stethoscope over artery and deflate the cuff gently and slowly	To maintain control over artery and control rate of deflation
Feel or listen for systolic blood pressure when Korotkoff (thudding) sound first felt or heard Diastolic blood pressure is when Korotkoff sound disappears	Ensures accurate reading obtained
Dooument the recording	Record accurately the reading and compare with previous recordings
Remove equipment and clean Ensure patient is comfortable	Reduces risk of cross-infection

PROCEDURE: PULSE OXIMETRY	
Action	**Rationale**
Explain and discuss with the patient and obtain consent	Ensures patient understanding and consent obtained is informed and valid
Ensure patient is warm and comfortable	Ensures peripheral circulation Cold and poor peripheral circulation interferes with reading
Wash and dry hands thoroughly Ensure equipment clean and working	Minimises cross-infection Ensures equipment suitable for use
Place probe as direct per instructions on suitable area, e.g., finger	Corrects function as per instruction
Switch on machine and allow it to calibrate	Ensures probe ready to detect reading
Document recording and report any abnormality, e.g., confusion, disorientation	Ensures patient problems communicated Ensures sufficient signal, correct saturation rate
Once complete remove probe, clean equipment and return to original place	Minimises risk of cross-infection

PROCEDURE: NEUROLOGICAL OBSERVATION

Glasgow coma score assesses the level of consciousness by monitoring: the patient's ability to open their eyes; motor and verbal response; vital signs and limb movement. The score ranges between three and 15, with 15 indicating a normal level and a score less than eight indicating deep coma. Any deterioration in the score indicates patient' consciousness level is deteriorating so needs to be reported immediately.

Action	Rationale
Tell the patient what is happening Provide them with instructions, e.g., open their eyes Ensure room is dimly lit when assessing pupil response Shine torch from side to side in one eye at a time to ascertain: size; quality; shape of pupils; reaction to light and intensity of reaction, i.e., sluggish, absent	If unable to open eyes indicates damage to the optic nerve and/or occulomotor nerve responsible for eyelid movement; swelling; trauma Important to identify any abnormality, e.g., cataracts, drugs or any medication patient may have had (atropine dilate pupils; opiates constrict pupils) Responses range from spontaneous eye opening to eyes not opening Pupil size should be 2–5 mm in diameter Inequality is a sign of raised intracranial pressure Different sized pupils indicate brain damage
Ask patient a series of questions, e.g., where are they?	Assesses if patient is aware of their surroundings Responses range from orientation to no response If unable to speak may be due to damage to speech centre in brain
Ask patient to squeeze your hands in their hands and release Ask them to push their feet against your hands	Assessing response of limbs Response ranges from obeying all commands to no response Detects extent of damage to motor cortex Releasing demonstrates a higher level of functioning in which the brain carries out the instruction, as opposed to being a primitive reflex response
Record vital sign: temperature, respiratory rate, pulse rate and blood pressure	Due to damage to thermoregulatory centre in the brain Good indicator of functioning brain stem. Monitoring respiratory rate and pattern is essential as it may be due to rise in intracranial pressure or Cushing's reflex (if respiratory rate falls) Raised BP and reduced pulse indicates raised intracranial pressure

References

Auken, S and Crawford, B (1998) Neurological Observations. In Guerro, D (ed.) *Neuro Oncology for Nurses.* Whurr, London.

Baille, L (ed) (2001) *Developing Nursing Skills.* Arnold, London.

British Hypertension Society (2004) Guidelines for Management of Hypertension: Report of the Fourth Working Party of the British Hypertension Society, *Journal of Human Hypertension* 18: 139–185.

Brooker, C and Waugh, A (2007) *Foundations of Nursing Practice, Fundamentals of Holistic Care.* Mosby, Edinburgh.

Carlson, DS (2002) Neurologic Clinical Assessment. In L. Urden, M. Lough and K. Stacy (eds) *Critical Care Nursing: Diagnosis and Management,* 4th edn. Mosby, St Louis.

Chandler, T (2001) Oxygen Administration, *Paediatric Nursing* 13(8): 37–42.

Cuddy, M (2004) The Effects of Drugs on Thermoregulation, *Advanced Practice in Acute Critical Care* 15(2): 238–253.

Dawes, E et al. (2007) Monitoring and Recording Patient's Neurological Observations, *Nursing Standard* 22(10): 40–45.

Dawson, D and Shah, S (2006) Neurological Care. In Sheppard M and Wright, M (eds) *Principles and Practice of High Dependency Nursing,* 2nd edn. Elsevier, Edinburgh.

Dougherty, L and Lister, S (2006) *The Royal Marsden Hospital Manual of Clinical Nursing Procedure,* 6th edn. Blackwell Publishing, London.

Dougherty, L and Lister, S (2008) *The Royal Marsden Hospital Manual of Clinical Nursing Procedure Student Edn,* 7th edn. Blackwell Publishing, London.

European Society of Hypertension-European Society of Cardiology Guidelines for the Management of Arterial Hypertension Guidelines Committee (2003), *Journal of Hypertension* 21: 1011–1053.

Evans, D et al. (1994) *Vital Signs.* The Joanna Briggs Institute, Australia.

Field, D (2000) Respiratory Care. In Sheppard, M and Wright, M (eds) *Principles and Practice of High Dependency Nursing.* Balliere Tindall, Edinburgh.

Frawley, P (1990) Critical Care. Neurological Observation, *Nursing Times* 86(35): 29–34.

Grant, J et al. (1990) A Method of Validating Nursing Diagnosis Advances, *Nursing Science* 12(3): 65–74.

Helms, P (2000) The Respiratory System. In Hoddard, D (ed.) *Care Paediatrics and Child Health.* Churchill Livingstone, London.

Hickey, JV (1997) *The Clinical Practice of Neurological and Neurosurgical Nursing,* 4th edn. Lippincott, New York.

Hickey, JV (2002) *The Clinical Practice of Neurological and Neurosurgical Nursing,* 5th edn. JB Lippincott, Philadelphia.

Hickey, J (2003) Neurological Assessment. In Hickey J (ed.) *The Clinical Practice of Neurological and Neurosurgical Assessment,* 5th edn. Lippincott Williams and Wilkins, Philadelphia.

Higgins, D (2005) Pulse Oximetry, *Nursing Times* 101(06): 34–35.

Howell, M (2002) The Correct Use of Pulse Oximetry in Measuring Oxygen Status, *Professional Nurse* 17(7): 416–418.

Kaye, AH (2005) *Neurological Assessment and Examination Essential Neurosurgery,* 3rd edn. Blackwell Publishing, Oxford.

Marieb, EM and Hoehn, K (2007) *Human Anatomy and Physiology*. Pearson Benjamin Cummings, San Francisco.

Marini, JJ and Wheeler, AP (2006) *Critical Care Medicine: The Essentials*. Lippincott Williams and Wilkins, Philadelphia.

McCance, K and Heuther, S (2006) *Pathophysiology: The Biological Basis for Disease in Adults and Children,* 5th edn. Mosby, St Louis.

Neno, R (2005) Hypothermia: Assessment, Treatment and Prevention, *Nursing Standard* 19(20): 47–52.

NICE (2003) *Head Injury: Triage, Assessment, Investigation and Early Measurement of Head Injury in Infants, Children and Adults,* Clinical Guidance 4. NICE, London.

NICE (2007) *CG56: Head Injury Observation Proforma and GCS* (online). NICE, London.

NMC (2007) *Guidance for the Introduction of the Essential Skills Clusters for Pre-Registration Nursing Programmes.* NMC, London.

O'Brien, E et al. (2001) ABC of Hypertension Blood Pressure Part IV – Automated Sphygmomanomotery: Self Blood Pressure Measurement, *British Journal of Medicine* 322: 531–636.

O'Brien, E et al. (2003) European Society of Hypertension Recommendations for Conventional, Ambulatory and Home Blood Pressure Measurement, *Journal of Hypertension* 21: 821–848.

Palmer, R and Knight, J (2006) Assessment of Altered Conscious Level in Clinical Practice, *British Journal of Nursing* 15(22): 1255–1259.

Petrie, JR (2003) Blood Pressure Measurement in Diabete: Theory and Practice, *British Journal of Diabetes and Vascular Disease*, 3(4): 258–261.

Shah, S (1999) Neurological Assessment, *Nursing Standard* 13(22): 49–56.

Stewart, N (1996) Neurological Observations, *Professional Nurse* 11(6): 377–378,

Thibodeau, G and Patton, KT (2007) *Anatomy and Physiology,* 6th edn. Mosby Elsevier, St Louis

Tortora, GJ and Derrickson, N (2008) *Principles of Anatomy and Physiology,* 12th edn. J. Wiley and Sons Inc, New York.

Trim, J (2005) Monitoring Temperature, *Nursing Times* 101(20): 30–31.

Waterhouse, C (2005) The Glasgow Coma Scale and Other Neurological Observation, *Nursing Standard* 19(33): 56–64.

WHO/Inter Soc of Hypertension Guidelines for the Management of Hypertension Guidelines Subcommittee (1999) 17: 151–183.

Weber, J and Kelley, J (2003) *Health Assessment in Nursing,* 2nd edn. Lippincott Williams and Wilkins, Philadelphia.

Williams, B et al. (2004) Guidelines for Management of Hypertension: Report of the 4th Working Party of the British Hypertension Society – BHSIV, *Journal of Human Hypertension* 18: 139–185.

Wong, DL et al. (2001) *Wong's Essentials of Paediatric Nursing,* 6th edn. Mosby St Louis.

Woodrow, P (1999) Pulse Oximetry, *Nursing Standard* 13(42): 42–46.

Woodrow, P (2005) Assessing Respiratory Function in Older People, *Nursing Older People* 14(3): 27–28.

Woollens, S (1996) Temperature Measurement Devices, *Professional Nurse* 11(8): 541–547.

Yarrows, SA et al. (2000) Home Blood Pressure Monitoring, *Arch Intern Med* 160: 1252–1257.

www.bhsoc.org/pdfs/BHS_IV_Guidelines.pdf

www.attract.wales.nhs.uk

7

Hygiene Needs

Learning Outcomes

This chapter is designed to help you:

o   recognise the importance of patients' personal hygiene needs
o   become familiar with the basics of hair, nail, eye, ear and nose care
o   understand the basics of oral care including (a) the role of assessment and (b) the efficacy of various tools.

Introduction

Good hygiene care helps to provide patients with comfort, promote recovery and facilitate discharge from hospital. This chapter provides a step by step approach to hygiene, including oral care, and considers the role of an holistic approach.

The Importance of Hygiene Needs

DH (2003) views personal hygiene as a 'physical act of cleaning the body to ensure that the skin, hair and nails are maintained in the optimum condition'. NMC (2007) notes that students 'provide care (or make provisions) for those who are unable to maintain their own personal care'. Patients expect their needs to be met according to their individual and clinical needs. Meeting these needs may involve nurses in intimate care. Providing hygiene needs involves questions of health, social acceptability, cultural norms concerning cleanliness and odour, and self-presentation (through, for example, grooming). Such aspects of care are covered in the Essence of Care document (DH 2001), which aims at improving practice pertaining to hygiene needs.

When an individual becomes ill he or she may require a nurse to help maintain hygiene and 'maintain an acceptable level of cleanliness' (Young 1991). Patients may feel embarrassed over becoming dependent and requiring assistance with the intimate acts involved in meeting hygiene needs. However, providing such intimate care can promote the patient's comfort, sense of well-being and self esteem. It may also help to improve skin and muscle condition (e.g., by stimulating circulation through massage) and to meet the religious, cultural, familial and psychosocial needs of the patient (Cooper 1994).

There is a suggestion that there is a link between appearing attractive and hygiene needs which begins in childhood. As children develop physically, they tend to learn to gain self control, become aware of their own independence and move away from dependency upon their parents. As they do so, they often perceive a link between hygiene needs and personal attractiveness (Bordo et al. 1990, Wong et al. 2003). Social and cultural beliefs also develop over this period, variously influenced by parents, carers, peers and a wish to conform to social norms.

Consider the challenges presented by (1) a female patient from an ethnic minority group who may not want a male nurse to help meet her hygiene needs due to cultural beliefs and (2) an elderly female patient who may not want a man other than her husband to see her with little clothing on. Nurses therefore need to be sensitive to social, cultural, religious and ethnic beliefs and preferences and must respect them. Effective nursing involves more than following routines such as that for performing bed baths. It also involves recognising the need for holistic care and patient choice (Walsh and Ford 1990, Bolander 1994, Holland et al. 2003). Assessment of hygiene needs should therefore take into account such matters as the patient's usual routines, their abilities, beliefs and preferences. Patients should be involved and rapport developed to facilitate individualised care. An holistic assessment will also identify opportunities for health promotion and referral to the multidisciplinary team, encourage independence and respect the need for privacy and dignity while also acknowledging patient limitations. Limitations might include reduced motivation, weakness or tiredness, pain, perceptual or cognitive impairment, muscular or musculoskeletal impairment (as with Parkinson's disease, orthopaedic problems), or reduced mobility (e.g., infusions or drains).

Overall, such assessment will enable the nurse to. assess the level of assistance required to maintain and promote personal hygiene; plan and negotiate hygiene needs for the patient; undertake observations of the patient's physical well being; use appropriate interpersonal communication skills; carry out appropriate interventions; and evaluate the effectiveness of care given. It will seek to facilitate access to a safe environment (the bathroom), use of the patient's own toiletries and an adherence to bath times and routines. Goals will be realistic and achievable and will recognise the specific needs of teenagers, older people and patients with learning disabilities (Hoeffer et al. 1997, Cambridge and Carnaby 2000, Lentz 2003).

Poor assessment of or provision for a patient's personal hygiene needs may result in a number of problems. These include: the patient's loss of independence; pressure sores; an increased infection rate; reduced range of movement; antisocial odours; infestations; patient's distress; delayed discharge home; and increased costs in patient care. Meeting a patient's personal hygiene needs is an integral part of the nurse's role: it allows the nurse to demonstrate a range of skills including assessment, communication and observational skills. The development of rapport with the patient allows the nurse to respond to individual needs and preferences. This facilitates fair and anti-discriminatory practice (NMC 2008).

Holistic Approach to Hygiene Needs

It is important to ensure that a focus on washing does not neglect the need for specific aspects such as hair, mouth and perineal/perianal care.

The perianal area requires meticulous care, because of the large colonies of bacteria living in or around this area. Warm water and disposable wipes need to be available. Such care is particularly important for patients prone to infections, pressure sores, diarrhoea and urinary tract infection (UTI). Care needs to be taken to ensure that the patient does not feel embarrassment or humiliation and that their dignity and privacy is respected. A dignified and professional approach is required from the nurse, supported by informed consent from the patient (NMC 2008).

LEARNING ACTIVITY 7.1

Reflect on your experience of assisting a patient with his or her hygiene needs.

- How do you feel when providing such care?
- How do you think your patient feels?

Soaps, lotions and talcs can cause irritation and infection of the mucous membranes, so warm water alone should be used to avoid irritating the mucous membranes and causing irritation or infection. During the development of male infants, the foreskin separates from the penis: it softens and becomes retractable by the age of two, making washing this area easier. Before this age, retraction of the foreskin should be avoided.

For babies, a sponge bath is suggested, as daily immersion is unnecessary. Immediately after a bath, the baby should be dried and wrapped since its body is unable to regulate temperature and so can lose heat rapidly. With young children, encourage their participation according to their age, supervise them while in the bath and do not leave them there unattended. Adolescents should be able to meet their own hygiene needs and at this particularly sensitive time of their body's development it is especially important to allow for and promote their independence. Among the older population the protective function of the skin begins to deteriorate, resulting in fragile skin, less oil and moisture production and a decrease in elasticity. With these patients, therefore, avoid excessive use of soap, moisturise after bathing, avoid using talc and continue to promote their independence.

REFER TO PROCEDURE: PERSONAL HYGIENE

Hair Care

Hair care has physical and also psychological effects as it is connected with patients' sense of self esteem. Brushing hair keeps it clean by removing dead epithelial cells and dust from the hair and scalp, especially if dandruff is present. Hair can reflect the state of a patient's health. Dirty scalp and hair result in discomfort and odour. Providing hair care can be easily achieved by assessing the patient's level of activity (i.e., identifying what they can do for themselves) and their condition (considering, for example, whether the patient suffers from alopecia hair loss due to cancer treatment or hormonal changes). Alopecia in women and children especially can affect their physical, psychological and social attractiveness, so sensitivity and a skilled approach is required. Use a neutral pH shampoo and refer the patient to a surgical appliance officer or hairdresser to discuss choices and the wearing of a wig (Dougherty and Lister 2008).

If the patient is mobile their hair should be washed while having a shower, as unkempt hair can become greasy (due to an accumulation of dried sweat and sebum if not washed). If the patient has restricted movement, move the patient to the end of the bed and hang their head over the edge of the bed or have a bowl at the end of the bed and wash their hair here – though this is inappropriate for those with a head, neck or spinal injury. Dry hair with a towel: if hairdryers are used they need to be checked for safety first.

Infants' hair should be shampooed daily to prevent **seborrhoea**. It is important to ensure that the water and environment are warm, as infants are susceptible to the cold. For infestations such as head lice, the school nurse or Health Visitor can provide treatment in the form of a free prescription to treat the infestation with, for example, medicated shampoo. A non-chemical approach involving the removal of head lice before they have begun to spread or reproduce, is adopted through shampooing and conditioning the hair twice weekly and combing wet hair with a fine-toothhead plastic comb. However, Roberts et al. (2000) suggest that the chemical approach remains the most effective approach overall when treating head lice.

Facial Hair

Shaving is best completed after bathing, when the skin is softer. An electric shaver can provide a safe, convenient method of shaving men with facial hair growth who are prone to bleeding (for example, those on anticoagulant therapy or who have a clotting disorder). If wet shaving is preferred, wet the face, apply shaving cream until a lather is formed and shave using small, firm strokes in the direction of the hair growth over taut skin. Rinse the razor frequently and shave the face before the neck. On completion of the shave, wash the face with water, dry the face thoroughly and use aftershave or cream as preferred by the patient. Pat the cream or aftershave and avoid rubbing the face to prevent skin irritation.

With frail or debilitated patients, gentle wiping or washing of facial hair after meals removes any food debris. It is important to adhere to cultural and religious beliefs, as some cultures and religions do not allow hair to be cut or facial hair to be shaved on a daily basis. Instead, trim a beard or moustache to maintain a well groomed appearance.

REFER TO PROCEDURE: FACIAL SHAVING

With women with facial hair, identify the cause of the facial hair (for example, drugs, reduced oestrogen levels after the menopause) as it can have psychological effects for the patient (e.g., embarrassment). Plucking or shaving is not recommended as it encourages quicker regrowth of the hair. Instead depilatory creams, waxing or bleaching may be advised, while electrolysis may be considered as a permanent solution for the removal of facial hair.

Nail Care

Nail beds can be used to indicate general health status as the shape, colour and condition can be easily observed. Nail care is important to ensure bacteria does not enter the nail bed and cause an infection. If bacteria are allowed to do so, the nails can become a source from which bacteria multiply, while the nails dry out and the patient bites their nails, thereby transferring bacteria buried on the surface of the nail into the mouth (Richardson, 2008). Toenails are more problematic because of the difficulty for older patients of reaching the feet, while they may also have difficulty maintaining foot care because the ageing process can cause the thickening of nails and skin and calluses can form.

Nail and foot care therefore require special attention so as to avoid pain and infection. Feet should be cleaned and dried between the toes to avoid fungal infections. This is best achieved after showering, taking a bath or after the feet have been soaked in a bowl of water, as this process allows the nails to soften. A nail brush can remove obvious matter and dead skin while the nails should be dried thoroughly for the aforementioned reasons.

Nail trimming must be performed by a professional manicurist or podiatrist using sterile equipment and to prevent infection from being spread. This is especially pertinent for those patients with an underlying medical condition such as diabetes or circulatory impairment because if the skin is inadvertently cut, it can allow an infection to enter the bloodstream, delay wound healing and potentially result in an amputation.

Special attention is therefore required when cleaning the feet and inbetween the toes to avoid fungal infections occurring (Geraghty 2005). However, powders and creams are available to treat infections, odours and moisturise the feet, while diabetics should be referred to the chiropodist for foot care and cutting toe nails, as poor peripheral circulation can result in skin breakdown and delayed skin healing. Those wearing thromboembolitic device (TED) stockings should also have their feet cleaned regularly and TED stockings renewed, according to trust policy. Patients should be encouraged to wear correctly fitting shoes that do not restrict or rub the feet causing corns or calluses, avoid walking barefoot (which can result in injury or an infection), exercise the feet to maintain circulation and for cold feet wear warm socks or use an extra blanket where necessary. Heat pads and hot water bottles should be avoided as they can result in burns.

Eye Care

Blinking and tears keep the eyes clean and moist while awake, but this ability is lost in unconscious patients, resulting in the cornea being at risk of damage. Eye care can and should form part of the hygiene routine when washing the face. Eye care is provided for a number of reasons – to remove any discharge and crusts from the eye, preventing infection being spread from one eye to another eye, or damage to the eye itself, prior to eye drop instillation, soothing eye irritation, preventing corneal damage or abrasion in the unconscious or sedated patient, lubricants keeping closed eyes from being damaged, newborns, and those having had eye surgery require attention for the aforementioned reasons. Other reasons for providing eye care are: relieving pain and discomfort; preventing and treating any infection; preventing further injury; detecting disease at an early stage; maintaining contact lens and care for the false eye prosthesis (Ashurst 1997, Cunningham and Gould 1998, Boyd-Monk 2005, Stollery et al. 2005).

An aseptic technique is required when providing eye care. The patient should be lying down or sitting with their head tilted and chin pointing backwards, making for easy access to the eyes and patient comfort (Stollery et al. 2005). A good light source facilitates assessment. Therefore, position the light above and behind the nurse instead of directly into the patient's eye, as this is extremely uncomfortable and can damage the delicate structures of the eye. Clean the eye with normal saline and gauze to prevent infection and keep the eyes moist.

Ears and Nose Care

The ears and nose should also be cleaned when meeting the patient's hygiene needs as deposits can result in impairment and reduced patency. Clean the ears and nose with warm water and a flannel behind and around the ears, and towel dry. *Do not* insert anything into the ears except a tympanic thermometer or otoscope as anything foreign can potentially damage the eardrum. Do not insert anything into the nose as this can injure the mucosa.

Patients receiving enteral feeding and oxygen therapy also require strict nasal care to avoid excessive drying and excoriation of the air passages. Clean the ears and nose with warm water, cotton wool or gauze, dry with a towel and apply a water-based lubricant to prevent discomfort and to maintain moisture to the nasal mucosa. Gently clean around piercings with warm water and cotton wool or gauze and dry thoroughly.

Oral Hygiene Needs

The mouth is involved in eating and drinking, tasting, breathing and communicating. If the mouth is affected in anyway, this may cause discomfort, loss of appetite, difficulty in speaking and can have a psychological impact on the patient. White (2004) has noted that oral care is often overlooked as an aspect of care. An assessment as recommended within the Essence of Care document (DH 2001) will provide a baseline for planning, implementing and evaluating individualised care.

Providing mouth care has physical and psychological functions important to individuals and maintaining their health and well being. It can help to moisten and clean the mouth, remove unpleasant tastes and freshen the breath. Simply brushing teeth can help to ease a dry mouth and remove any bad taste in the mouth. Maintaining a clean and comfortable oral cavity also helps patients to recover, reduces the risk of their health declining, aids communication and helps to maintain their dignity.

Damage to the mouth, be it due to lack of basic care, disease or treatment, may cause multiple problems and reduce the quality of life (White 2000, Miller and Kearney 2001, Borbasi et al. 2002, Sonis et al. 2004). This is noted by Freer (2000), who stated that all patients, from the ambulant to the unconscious, need oral care and that its provision has enormous holistic impacts on the individual. For infants and toddlers, dental care should begin once the first tooth appears due to dental caries occurring during these formative years and should be practised after each feed or meal. A soft paediatric toothbrush moistened with water and then toothpaste applied should be adopted at about 18 months of age. At two-to-three years of age the child should be introduced to the dentist and regular visits should be arranged for dental advice and monitoring. As part of this process, fluoride is required to prevent dental caries and this should continue throughout childhood, along with brushing teeth between meals and limiting the intake of sugary foods or drinks. This should continue into adulthood where education, support, regular oral assessment and use of oral equipment and agents are required.

LEARNING ACTIVITY 7.2

You are looking after a four year old child in a day nursery who has just had lunch. The child needs their teeth cleaning.

Reflect upon comfort, dignity and feelings of the child when cleaning the teeth. How would you evaluate the care given and decide what to change next time?

There is evidence to suggest that mouth care is required to keep the mucosa clean, soft, moist, intact and prevent infection, keep the lips clean, soft, moist and intact, remove food debris, alleviate pain, discomfort, enhance oral intake, prevent halitosis and freshen breath (Cooley 2002). However, there is a lack of research regarding the frequency of mouth care being provided. Roberts (2000a) recommends the use of an effective oral assessment tool to ensure an early detection of problems. Nurses also need to consider the patient's specific needs – especially children with difficulties such as Down's Syndrome or cleft palate, teenagers with braces who need specific advice regarding oral care, and the older person with dentures. For instance, frequent mouth care should be provided, e.g., four-hourly oral care will reduce the potential for infection from micro-organisms, while two-hourly oral care will reduce mouth care problems and ensure patient comfort, while hourly oral care is required for those patients who are receiving oxygen therapy, mouth breathing, are unconscious or have an infected mouth (Krishnasamy 1995).

LEARNING ACTIVITY 7.3

When providing mouth care to your patient consider the feelings involved in such intimate care.

- When cleaning dentures, how do you feel?
- How do you think your patient feels?

Mouth washes should only be used two to three times a day, depending upon individual assessments. Further research is required regarding the frequency of oral care for each clinical area (McNeill 2000). An assessment is required to plan effective care (Eilers 2004, Sonis et al. 2004, Jaroneski 2006, Quinn et al. 2007) as this will provide baseline data of the mouth (i.e., is it dry), identify whether there are any infections, enable the nurse to monitor response to therapy and identify any new problems that may arise (e.g., infections, inflammations). It also identifies patients who are nil by mouth (NBM), on a restricted diet, receiving oxygen or who suffer from a dry mucous membrane (Holmes and Mountain 1993). An assessment also helps identify poor oral hygiene. There may be a number of causes, for example vomiting or nausea; dehydration; poor nutrition; fasting; poor salivary production; oral tumours or surgery; ear, nose, throat (ENT) surgery; or poor oral care generally. All of this can contribute to problems concerning pain, ulcers, infections, bleeding, difficulties with communicating, swallowing, taste and stomatitis resulting in mucous membrane damage, reduced salivary function, or a dirty or a coated tongue indicating a potential fungal infection.

Assessment tools provide some indication of how often the oral cavity should be cleaned and help to identify and plan nursing interventions. Holmes and Mountain (1993) evaluated three oral assessment tools for reliability, validity and clinical usefulness and found the Oral Assessment Guide by Eilers et al. (2004) to be the preferred assessment tool. However, Coleman (2000) and Evan (2001) stated that assessment tools were not in common use as the reliability was dependent upon the same nurse doing the assessment on each occasion. Freer (2004) provides an example of an oral assessment tool and care plan that could be used (see pp. 96–100).

When providing mouth care, toothbrushes and toothpaste should be used to clean teeth (Xavier 2000, Pearson and Hutton 2002). Foam sticks are ineffective in removing debris (Clay 2000) but are useful for refreshing the mouth and can cause less trauma when oral bleeding occurs (Lee et al. 2001). Pearson (1996) found that toothbrushes were more effective in removing dental plaque. Encourage patients to maintain their own oral hygiene needs if they are able to do so.

REFER TO PROCEDURE: MOUTH CARE

LEARNING ACTIVITY 7.4

Alex has suffered a serious head injury. Alex has now been discharged from ITU to a general ward and needs total care. As the nurse allocated to care for Alex, you have to assess Alex's needs. No record of oral assessment or hygiene has been recorded in the nursing notes and you are required to assess Alex's mouth.

1   How would you assess Alex's mouth?
2   What tools would you use?
3   How would you evaluate the care given and decide what to change next time?

ORAL ASSESSMENT TOOL

Name _____   Ward _____   Hospital Number _____

Tongue		Teeth or dentures		Saliva		Mucous membranes		Lips	
Pink and moist	1	Clean	1	Present/watery	1	Pink and moist	1	Smooth/moist	1
Coated	2	Plaque/debris in localised areas	2	Thick	2	Reddened/coated	2	Dry/cracked	2
Shiny/red	3	Plaque/debris along gum line	3	Insufficient	3	White areas	3	Bleeding	3
Blistered/cracked	4	Ill fitting dentures/caries	4	Absent	4	Ulcerated/bleeding	4	Ulcerated	4

Mental status		Pain		Nutritional intake		Other factors	
Alert	0	Pain free	0	Good	0		
Apathetic	1	Fear of pain	1	Inadequate diet	1	Steroid therapy	1
Sedated	2	Intermittent	2	Fluids only	2	Diabetes	2
Uncooperative	3	Pain on movement	3	Enteral	3	Oxygen therapy	3
Unconscious	4	Uncontrolled	4	No intake	4	Mouth breathing	4

SCORE   5–9: LOW RISK;   PLAN 6A
SCORE 10–17: RISK OF/EVIDENCE OF DRY MOUTH;   PLAN 6B
SCORE 18–28: RISK OF/EVIDENCE OF THRUSH;   PLAN 6C
SCORE 29–31: RISK OF/EVIDENCE OF SORE MOUTH/TONGUE;   PLAN 6D
SCORE 32–36: RISK OF/EVIDENCE OF ULCERATED MOUTH;   PLAN 6E

Re-evaluate every other day.

ORAL ASSESSMENT: CONTINUATION SHEET

Name ———————— Ward ———————— Hospital Number ————————

Date	Time	Assessment score	Risk of . . .	Or evidence of . . .	Plans of care	Assessed by	Review due

©Freer 04

ORAL HYGIENE PLANS (Tick plans in use)

PLAN OF CARE 6A: FOUNDATION CARE THROUGHOUT

Nursing Action	Rationale
Brush teeth/dentures twice daily using toothbrush and toothpaste. If not possible, use foam sticks soaked in Corsodyl.	To remove plaque/debris from teeth and gums (1). A toothbrush and toothpaste is the most effective tool for cleaning the mouth (2, 11, 12). Foam sticks used with Corsodyl can reduce plaque (3, 12).
Soak dentures overnight in cold water/proprietary denture cleaner and brush.	Inhibits formation of plaque and oral infections (4, 12).
Reassess every other day or sooner if condition changes and provide advice/encouragement to patient/carer to participate.	To evaluate efficacy of current plan of care (4, 5, 9). This is pivotal in reducing the risk of further problems (11, 13).

Plan of Care 6B: DRY MOUTH (Xerostomia)

Offer cold water/soda water, at least 30 ml per hour. Use foam sticks if preferred or cannot swallow.	Provides temporary but refreshing relief. More effective if fluids are given regularly (4). Foam sticks are effective in moistening oral mucosa (3).
Offer crushed ice to suck.	Provides a temporary cooling effect (4).
Offer unsweetened pineapple chunks/juice to suck if available.	Pineapple contains ananase, an enzyme which cleans the mouth (6, 12).
Suggest the regular use of lip balm.	Can prevent cracking of lips. Caution with petroleum-based when using oxygen (4, 7, 12).
Consider with medical staff whether artificial saliva in conjunction with the above is appropriate, e.g., Oral Balance gel (16, 17).	The range of artificial saliva's on the market provide a variety of actions; oral tissue protection, stimulation of salivary flow, anti-bacterial protection (8, 12, 16, 17).

Plan of Care 6C: THRUSH (Candidiasis)

Inform medical staff immediately to consider the use of antifungal medication, e.g., Nystatin, Fluconazole. Ensure review of medication effectiveness occurs.	Early treatment of infection can minimise symptoms and prevent erosion of mucosa and spread to other parts of the GI tract (4,7).
Brush teeth/dentures after each meal.	Prevents organisms being trapped in gums, dentures or teeth (8, 12).
Soak dentures overnight in Corsodyl.	To prevent reinfection of the oral mucosa (9).

Plan of Care 6D: SORE MOUTH

Brush teeth and tongue twice daily with a soft toothbrush soaked in Difflam.	To aid lifting of debris (10). A soft toothbrush can prevent trauma and reduce infection risk (2, 11, 12). Difflam contains a local anaesthetic (1).
Offer fizzy drinks/soda water hourly.	Effervescence aids the lifting of debris (10).
Consider Vitamin C effervescent tablets with medical staff.	Effervescence aids the lifting of debris (10).
Offer pineapple chunks to suck/chew.	Contains ananase, an enzyme which helps to clean the tongue (6, 12).

Plan of Care 6B: ULCERATED MOUTH

Remove dentures and soak in fresh cold water (change water daily).	Dentures may be too painful to wear. If exposed to heat or left to dry, dentures can become warped and ill fitting (1, 4).
Discuss with medical staff a prescription for a local anaesthetic mouthwash/gel.	Can offer relief (and coating initially) so enabling oral intake to continue (6, 7).

© Freer 04

Water can be used for mouth care, while artificial saliva may be more beneficial than water (Duxberry et al. 1989). Mouthwash tablets dry out the mucosa, if used long term. Pieces of pineapple contain a protein-digesting enzyme that cleans the tongue so chewing or sucking them should be encouraged. They also have a refreshing effect and stimulate salivation. Lemon and glycerine should not be used as glycerine dehydrates the oral mucosa and the acidity of lemon juice damages tooth enamel (Bowsher 1999, Rattenbury et al. 1999). Lip balm and soft paraffin moisturises the lips and prevents them from cracking by forming an oil film that reduces water loss through evaporation. This has added importance for the older person where oral mucosa becomes dry due to reduced saliva production and infrequent fluid intake.

Cleanse dentures overnight to prevent thrush. Use the patient's own denture container, a sterilising tablet and rinse under water, with a soft toothbrush and toothpaste. Toothpaste with fluoride is available, though over-exposure to fluoride results in fluorosis in children. Good oral hygiene involves cleaning the teeth with a toothbrush and toothpaste after meals; using five millilitres of chlorhexidine diluted in one hundred millilitres of water four times a day, rinsed for one minute before expelling.

Summary

Providing patient hygiene needs is often straightforward and allows the nurse to build a rapport with their patient, reduce any barriers between patient and healthcare professional and assess, treat, diagnose and plan care effectively. It therefore promotes holistic and individualised care. It is essential to continue to assess and review, to communicate with the patient, promote independence and self esteem, and maintain the patient's dignity. In the ever changing world of nursing, hygiene should not be reduced to a ritualistic part of the nurse's role – especially given the focus on hygiene needs within the Essence of Care document (DH 2001).

PROCEDURE: PERSONAL HYGIENE	
Action	Rationale
Assess the patient's needs considering their cultural and religious needs Involve the patient and family	Plan care Encourages participation and independence
Explain what is occurring and obtain consent	Ensures patient understanding and ensures consent is informed
Offer the opportunity of bedpan/commode/ toilet/urinal prior to hygiene needs being met	Minimises disruption while washing Prevents discomfort
Collect equipment, e.g., bed linen, towel(s), flannel/disposable wipe(s), toiletries, clean clothing, bowl and water	Minimises disruption and time away from the patient Disposable wipes reduces risk of cross-infection

(Cont'd)

Action	Rationale
Ensure bed area is draught free, private and free of excess equipment by closing door/drawing curtains	Maintains safe environment Promotes privacy and dignity
Wash and dry hands thoroughly Wear disposable apron	Minimises risk of cross-infection
Assist patient to remove clothing, cover them with a blanket/towel having folded back bed linen	Maintains privacy, dignity and minimises embarrassment Minimises body exposure to a cold environment thereby not reducing body temperature
Check if soap used on face, neck, ears Wash, rinse and dry thoroughly	Promotes cleanliness and independence Minimises the time body exposed to cold environment
Wash, rinse and dry thoroughly trunk of body and arms using toiletries as preferred, taking care of drips, drains and dressings in situ Observe skin condition for sores, infections, inflammation, bruising	Promotes well being, cleanliness and reduces risk of cross-infection Identifies potential risk of pressure sores and/or any pressure sores developing
Change water to wash genitalia Inform patient and encourage independence by encouraging patient to wash here Also gain consent to wash the genitalia using separate disposable wipes and dry thoroughly wearing gloves If a catheter is in situ wash around the urethral meatus and away from the genetalia while wearing gloves. Rinse and dry thoroughly In circumcised men, draw back the foreskin to wash and if uncircumcised, do not retract the foreskin	Promotes cleanliness, well being and reduces risk of cross-infection Promotes independence and participation in care
Change water and gloves Assist men to shave	Promotes positive body image Maintains cleanliness Preserves privacy and dignity
Assist with dressing and change bed linen If patient still in bed two nurses required	Reduces unnecessary activity for patient and nurse Maintains safety and safe manual handling
Ensure mouth care needs met so provide equipment, e.g., toothbrush, toothpaste,	Maintains oral hygiene and enhances comfort

Action	Rationale
bowls, cups of water and position the patient to facilitate this process	
Wash, dry and comb hair if requested hair care	Enhances patient comfort and positive body image
Remove, clean and dry equipment and return patient possessions, e.g., table, locker, call bell within easy reach Ensure patient comfort Open door/draw back the curtains	Maintains safe environment and promotes patient independence
Remove and dispose of apron and gloves as per trust policy Wash and thoroughly dry hands	Prevents cross-infection
Document all care and any changes	Provides a recorded documentation of care and facilitates communication

PROCEDURE: MOUTH CARE

Action	Rationale
Explain and discuss the procedure Gain consent	Ensures patient understanding and consent is informed and valid
Wash and dry hands thoroughly	Reduces the risk of infection
Obtain and prepare environment, e.g., close the door/draw curtains; have toothbrush/toothpaste, receiver, water, towel available	Maximises efficacy and minimises risk of microbial contamination Promotes patient participation
Inspect patient mouth, lips, tongue, gums	Examine for change in condition regarding moisture, cleanliness, infection, bleeding gums
Using soft, small toothbrush and toothpaste brush teeth, gums, tongue at 45 degree angle, moving back and forth, and with a vibrating motion, if the patient is unable to do so Clean the biting surfaces in short strokes	Removes debris from the teeth, tongue, gums Brushing stimulates gingival tissues to maintain tone and prevent circulatory stasis; loosens and removes debris on and between teeth and gums Reduces growth of micro-organisms Minimises risk of plaque formation and dental caries

(Cont'd)

Action	Rationale
Allow and encourage patient to rinse mouth vigorously and empty into a receiver, with towel close to hand If patient unable to do this or brush teeth, consider using foam sticks to freshen mouth, gums, mucosa	Rinsing removes loosened debris Toothpaste freshens mouth Foam sticks are ineffective in removing debris; only freshens the mouth and provides moisture
Apply lubricant to dry lips	Increases patient comfort, well being and prevents further tissue damage
Clean dentures (if worn) with a toothbrush and toothpaste, rinse well and return to patient after being soaked overnight in a denture pot with a denture cleanser	Removes debris Some denture cleaners have an abrasive effect, attracts plaque and encourages bacterial growth Reduces risk of re-infecting mouth
Discard mouth, wash items, clean and dry toothbrush thoroughly Wash and dry hands thoroughly	Prevents risk of contamination Reduces risk of cross-infection

PROCEDURE: FACIAL SHAVING

Action	Rationale
Explain and discuss procedure and obtain consent	Ensures patient understanding and consent is informed and valid
Ascertain patient preference for a shave, i.e., wet or dry shave	Individualises care
Wash and dry hands thoroughly Wear apron and gloves	Reduces and minimises cross-infection
Drape towel across patient chest and assess face for any sores or moles	Protection
Encourage patient to shave self If unable to do so apply cream/foam/soap to face and lather	Promotes independence
Using short strokes in the direction of the hair growth, shave face at cheeks down to the neck, pulling skin taut with free hand	Shaves in the direction of the growth of the whiskers
Rinse razor after each stroke and once shaved, rinse face with clean water and dry thoroughly Apply aftershave/cream/cologne	Promotes well being and cleanliness

Action	Rationale
Dispose of water/equipment and return personal items, e.g., toiletries to locker, call bell close to hand	Maintains safe environment
Remove gloves and apron as per trust policy	Minimises cross-infection
Document care given	Facilitates communication

References

Ashurst, S (1997) Nursing Care of the Mechanically Ventilated Patient in ICU: 1, *British Journal of Nursing* 6(8): 447–454.

Bolander, V (1994) *Sorenson and Luckmann's Basic Nursing: A Psychophysiologic Approach,* 3rd edn. Saunders, Philadelphia. Chapter 38.

Borbasi, S et al. (2002) More Than a Sore Mouth: Patients Experience of Oral Mucositis, *Oncology Nursing Forum* 29(7): 1051–1057.

Bordo, S et al. (1990) Reading the Slender Body. In Jacobus, M et al. *Body of Politics: Women and the Discourses of Science*. Routledge, London.

Bowsher, J et al. (1999) Oral Care, *Nursing Standard* 13(37): 31.

Boyd-Monk, H (2005) Bringing Common Eye Emergencies into Focus, *Nursing* 35(12): 46–51.

Cambridge, A and Carnaby, P (2000) *Making it Personal: Providing Intimate and Personal Care for People with Intellectual Disabilities*. Pavilion, Brighton.

Clay, M (2000) Oral Health in Older People, *Nursing Older People* 12(7): 21–26.

Coleman, P (2000) Improving Oral Healthcare for the Frail Elderly: A Review of Widespread Problems and Best Practices, *Geriatric Nursing* 23(4): 189–199.

Cooley, C (2002) Oral Health: Basic or Essential Care? *Cancer Nursing Practice* 1(3): 33–39.

Cooper, C (1994) Hygiene and the Client. In McMahon, A and Harding, J (eds) *Knowledge to Care*. Blackwell Scientific, Oxford.

Cunningham, C and Gould, D (1998) Eyecare for the Sedated Patient Undergoing Mechanical Ventilation: The Use of Evidence Based Care, *International Journal of Nursing Studies* 35: 32–40.

DH (2001) *Essence of Care*. DH, London.

DH (2003) *Winning Ways: Working Together to Reduce Healthcare Associated Infection in England*. DH, London.

Dougherty, L and Lister, S (2008) *The Royal Marsden Hospital Manual of Clinical Nursing Procedures Student Edition*, 7th edn. Wiley Blackwell, Oxford.

Duxberry, AJ et al. (1989) A Double Blind Cross Over Trial of a Mucin – Containing Artificial Saliva, *British Dental Journal* 166(4): 115–120.

Eilers, J (2004) Nursing Interventions and Supportive Care for the Prevention and Treatment of Oral Mucositis Associated with Cancer Treatment, *Oncology Nursing Forum* 31(4): 13–23.

Evan, G (2001) A Rationale for Oral Care, *Nursing Standard* 15(43): 33–36.

Freer, S (2000) Use an Oral Assessment Tool to Improve Practice, *Professional Nurse* 15(10): 635–637.

Freer, S (2004) *Oral Assessment Tool and Oral Hygiene Care Plans,* Nottingham University Hospital, NHS Trust Nottingham.

Geraghty, M (2005) Nursing the Unconscious Patient, *Nursing Standard* 20(1): 54–64.

Hoeffer, B et al. (1997) Reducing Aggressive Behaviour During Bathing Cognitively Impaired Nursing Home Residents, *Journal of Gerontology Nursing* 23(5): 16–23.

Holland, K et al. (2003) *Applying the Roper Logan Tierney Model in Practice.* Churchill Livingstone, Edinburgh.

Holmes, S and Mountain, T (1993) Assessment of Oral Status: Evaluation of Three Oral Assessment Guides, *Journal of Clinical Nursing* 2: 35–40.

Krishnasamy, M (1995) Oral Problems in Advanced Cancer, *European Journal of Cancer Care* 4: 173–177.

Jaroneski, LA (2006) The Importance of Assessment Rating Scales for Chemotherapy Induced Oral Mucositis, *Journal of Clinical Nursing* 2: 35–40.

Lee, J et al. (2001) An Audit of Oral Care Practice and Staff Knowledge in Hospital Palliative Care, *International Journal of Palliative Nursing* 7(8): 395–400.

Lentz, J (2003) Daily Baths: Torment or Comfort at End of Life? *Journal of Hospice Palliative Nursing* 5(1): 34–39.

McNeill, HE (2000) Biting Back at Poor Oral Hygiene, *Intensive and Critical Care Nursing* 16: 367–372.

Miller, M and Kearney, N (2001) Oral Care for Patients with Cancer: A Review of the Literature, *Cancer Nurse* 24(4): 241–254.

NMC (2007) *Guidance for the Introduction of the Essential Skills Clusters for Pre-Registration Nursing Programmes.* NMC, London.

NMC (2008) *The Code: Standards of Conduct, Performance and Ethics for Nurses and Midwives.* NMC, London.

Pearson, L (1996) A Comparison of the Ability of Foam Swabs and Toothbrushes to Remove Dental Plaque: Implications for Nursing Practice, *Journal of Advanced Nursing Practice* 23: 62–69.

Pearson, LS and Hutton, JL (2002) A Controlled Trial to Compare the Ability of Foam Sticks, Swabs and Toothbrushes to Remove Dental Plaque, *Journal of Advanced Nursing* 39(5): 480–489.

Quinn, B et al. (2007) Ensuring Accurate Oral Mucositis Assessment in the European Group for Blood and Marrow Transplantation Prospective Oral Mucositis Audit, *European Journal of Oncology Nursing* 11(Supplement): 10–18.

Rattenbury, N et al. (1999) Oral Assessment and Care for Inpatients, *Nursing Times* 95(49): 52–53.

Richardson, R (ed.) (2008) *Clinical Skills for Student Nurses Theory, Practice and Reflection.* Reflect Press, Devon.

Roberts, RJ et al. (2000) Comparison of Wet Combing with Malathion for Treatment of Head Lice in the UK: A Pragmatic Randomised Controlled Trial, *Lancet* 356: 540–544.

Roberts, J (2000a) Developing an Oral Assessment Tool and Intervention Tool for Older People 3, *British Journal of Nursing* 9(19): 2073–2078.

Sonis, S et al. (2004) Perspectives on Cancer Therapy-Induced Mucosal Injury: Pathogenesis Measurement Epidemiology and Consequences for Patients, *Cancer Supplement* 100(9): 1995–2025.

Stollery, R et al. (2005) *Opthalmic Nursing,* 3rd edn. Blackwell Publishing, Oxford.

Walsh, M and Ford, P (1990) *Nursing Rituals, Research and Rational Actions.* Butterworth-Heinneman, Oxford.

White, RJ (2000) Nurse Assessment of Oral Health: A Review of Practice and Education, *British Journal of Nursing* 9(5): 260–266.

White, R (2004) Oral Health Assessment: A Review of Current Practice. In White, R (ed.) *Trends in oral Healthcare.* Quay Books, Wiltshire, pp. 1–10.

Wong, DL et al. (2003) *Wong's Essentials of Paediatric Nursing,* 6th edn. Mosby, St Louis.

Xavier, G (2000) The Importance of Mouth Care in Preventing Infection, *Nursing Standard* 14(18): 47–51.

Young, L (1991) The Clean Fight, *Nursing Standard* 5(35): 54–55.

8

Nutritional and Hydrational Needs

Learning Outcomes

This chapter is designed to help you:

o   understand the principles of nutritional assessment and screening
o   consider what constitutes (a) malnutrition and (b) normal eating and drinking
o   understand the types of nutritional support required by patients
o   be aware of professional responsibilities regarding nutrition and feeding
o   understand hydration needs.

Introduction

Food is essential for life: it provides nutrients to sustain body functions and homeostasis. Eating is a basic human and social activity. Meal times may provide opportunities for families to sit down and eat together and ensure children eat a healthy balanced diet. Its importance is emphasised in the Essence of Care document (DH 2001), which states that patients should 'receive the care and assistance they require with eating and drinking'. However, food and nutrition have been identified by patients as an often unsatisfactory feature of the care provided by the National Health Service (NHS). Patients complain of a lack of choice and the poor taste and unattractive appearance of the food they have been provided with.

Nurses need to ensure that patients receive adequate nutrition and frequently need to help patients to eat and drink. Good nutrition is fundamental for health and promotes recovery from illness or injury. The NMC (2007) Essential Skills Clusters identify nutrition and fluid management as fundamental skills in which all nurses must be competent. In particular, nursing involves educating people regarding eating and drinking for optimum health. It also involves working with the multidisciplinary team (MDT) to promote hydration and nutrition.

Nutrition and hydration maintain **homeostasis**, allowing oxygen, nutrients and other metabolic substances to enter the cells and waste products to be excreted. Inadequate fluid and nutrient intake impedes recovery from illness, lengthens hospital stay and can lead to complications (for example, delayed wound healing, pressure sore development, weight loss, dehydration, poor oral hygiene, depression).

Nutritional Assessment and Screening

Nutritional assessment entails a detailed investigation to identify and quantify specific dietary problems (Bond 1997) in order to identify those at risk of **malnutrition** and those with poor nutritional status. Nutritional screening is the first line process of identifying patients who are already malnourished, or are at risk of malnourishment (Green and Watson 2005). Undertaking a nutritional assessment and screening as part of the admission process is therefore essential.

Many tools for nutritional assessment have been developed (Collier 2002, Devlin 2000, Ledsham and Gough 2000). BAPEN (2003), for example, launched a tool which could be used to screen for malnutrition in all clinical settings. Stratton et al. (2004), however, found a high prevalence of malnutrition in hospitalised patients (19–60 per cent) occurring, despite the use of screening tools such as the malnutrition universal screening tool (MUST). However, it is still important that a nutrition plan is developed to meet the needs of the patient based on assessment and screening.

Malnutrition may mean either over- or under-nutrition (Green and Watson 2005). Malnutrition is a condition that occurs when the body fails to receive appropriate nutrients. It may result from an inadequate or unbalanced diet, digestive difficulties, absorption problems, or a medical condition. The incidence of malnutrition in children admitted to hospital was estimated to be as high as 50 per cent, while 15 to 20 per cent admitted to a paediatric intensive care unit (PICU) (Huddleston et al. 1993) have been found to be malnourished.

Malnutrition is associated with numerous problems. They include weight loss, lower than normal growth, a bloated abdomen, changes in skin and hair (brittle nails, hair loss, dry scaly skin), impaired respiratory and cardiac function, decreased mobility due to muscle wasting, weak muscles, bone or joint pain (Lennard-Jones 1992), an increased risk of infection and delayed wound healing (Chandra 1990, Windsor et al. 1988), depression and lethargy (Brozek 1990). Malnutrition may jeopardise health in general and can delay recovery from illness and discharge from hospitality – and even increase mortality (Robinson et al. 1987, Sullivan 1992).

LEARNING ACTIVITY 8.1

While undertaking a paediatric placement a student was involved in the admission of a 10 year old girl who was admitted for minor surgery.

During the admission assessment the family stated they were Muslim and only ate halal food. This was recorded in the notes. The following day it was noted that the correct food was not present on the trolley. The staff nurse decided that as the parents were not present and the girl would not know the difference, gave her the food (even though it was not halal). The girl ate the food.

- What are the underlying issues here?
- What would you do if you came across a situation like this again?

Factors That May Prevent Normal Eating and Drinking

Nutrition is affected by several factors and it is the nurses' responsibility to identify those that increase the risk of nutritional problems occurring.

Box 8.1 Factors Affecting Normal Eating and Drinking

Inadequate cooking facilities
Budget
Food intake
Storage facilities
Lack of knowledge regarding a balanced diet
Poverty
Environment (access to the aforementioned)
Living and eating alone
Alcohol or substance abuse
Food preferences
Religious and cultural beliefs, e.g., Hindus not eating beef, Muslims eating halal meat
Mental health problems, e.g., depression
Physical problems, e.g., stroke, arthritis, chewing or swallowing difficulties may prevent patients from eating
Surgery
Nausea and vomiting
Gastrointestinal problems, e.g., anorexia, bulimia
Changes to the senses depress the taste buds so every meal tastes bland
Immobility
Poor manual dexterity (so provide utensils to help with eating)
Altered consciousness levels
Fluid or electrolyte imbalance
Chronic illness, e.g., renal or liver disease.

(Brooker and Waugh 2007)

Concern over food can have a psychological impact on patients, i.e., they may be left for lengthy periods of time without adequate intake, wondering when they may eat and whether the meal the patient receives will be sufficient and/or enough to 'fill them up'. This can result in a decrease in tissue mass and energy stores required for proper growth, can affect any age group across the lifespan and impede the ability to fight illness. An imbalance in bodily fluids and electrolytes may present itself as the patient becoming confused and there are many factors that contribute to this occurring.

Box 8.2 Factors Affecting Fluid and Electrolyte Imbalance

Poverty
Age
Fasting
Fluid imbalance due to diarrhoea and vomiting

(Cont'd)

Alcohol and caffeine drinks increases urine output and fluid depletion

Disability, i.e., learning disabilities, physical disabilities (may be unable to ask for a drink, chew, swallow, have poor muscle tone and posture difficulties)

Mental health problems, e.g., dementia, depression (may forget to drink/eat or if they have had a drink/eat resulting in fluid and electrolyte imbalance)

Immobility or lack of manual dexterity, e.g., arthritis, stroke, Parkinson's (hazardous due to difficulty holding a cup)

Dysphagia

Fear of incontinence

Drugs, e.g., diuretics

Abdominal pain

Social isolation.

(Brooker and Waugh 2007)

The factors listed above may result in weight loss starvation and nutritional deficiencies, an impaired immune system, post-operative complications, delayed recovery, delayed discharge and a need for nutritional support.

Nutritional Support

Dougherty and Lister (2006) defined nutritional support as 'any method of giving nutrients which encourages an optimal nutritional status'. It includes modifying the types of foods eaten, dietary supplementation, **enteral tube feeding** and **parenteral nutrition** (National Collaborating Centre for Acute Care 2006), while NICE (2006) defined nutritional support as 'methods to improve or maintain nutritional intake'. It has become an important therapeutic intervention for improving the outcomes of care for hospitalised patients (Marik et al. 2001). Nutritional support is required to prevent or rectify nutritional problems, e.g., failure to thrive, eating disorders, malnutrition, being NBM, bowel obstruction, surgery (head, neck, oesophagus), or increased metabolic rate (burns, major trauma) (Thomas 2001).

An assessment should be undertaken and include a consideration of the patient's physical appearance (for example, is the patient wearing loose-fitting clothing?), mobility, swallowing ability (i.e., lack of swallowing and gag reflex), whether there is a history (e.g., anorexia, bulimia) and whether there are pressure sores. Assess the mouth and teeth (are there, for example, any mouth ulcers, ill fitting dentures that make it difficult to eat?), the patient's mood and behaviour (for lethargy, poor concentration), bowel function (for constipation), urine output, BP (which will be hypertensive if overloaded, hypotensive if dehydrated), pulse (tachycardic due to hypovolaemia or overloaded with fluid), and fontanelles in babies (which should be level: sunken indicates dehydration, bulging indicates overloaded or raised intracranial pressure). If any of the difficulties are present, then provide aids and give encouragement. Ensure that a variety of drinks is available and that water jugs are changed regularly. Involve specialists such as dieticians and Speech and Language Therapists (SALT) wherever appropriate.

This need for nutritional support may also arise from the malfunction of the gastrointestinal tract, or the patient being NBM or unconscious. Nutritional support may take the form of enteral feeding or parenteral feeding. Enteral feeding is the passing of a tube via the nose into the stomach or jujenum (nasogastric tube) for short term feeding. For long term feeding a percutaneous endoscopic gastrostomy (PEG) tube is inserted directly into a patient's stomach via the abdominal wall and held in place by a balloon or flange. Other feeding routes include nasoduodenal or nasojejunal tubes being passed into the small intestine through the nose, oesophagus and stomach/jejunum. However, there is a risk of bacterial contamination, gastroenteritis or diarrhoea with enteral feeding so it is essential to follow the manufacturers' instructions and local policy whenever inserting the tube. It is then important to tailor enteral feeding to the individual patient's needs, to ensure the patient receives all the nutrients they require.

By making use of a functioning gastrointestinal tract in enteral feeding, the incidence of infection or contamination of the feed or cannulation site is reduced (Zainal 1994). Aspiration is a major risk as is inadequate nutrition and tube blocking, so flushing regularly with additional water is required to maintain hydration and keep the tube patent (Malik et al. 2004).

Liquid feed is either given through a fine tube being inserted via the nostril into the stomach (nasogastric feeding), directly into the stomach (gastrostomy or PEG feeding), or directly into the small bowel (jejunostomy feeding). A small bore nasogastric feeding tube is preferred rather than a wide bore tube because it allows normal swallowing, reduces the chance of phayngitis, rhinitis, mucosal erosion and is more comfortable and easier to tolerate (Payne-James et al. 2001). A wide bore tube is used to empty the stomach contents after surgery. The advantages are that this provides easy access and the tube is less likely to become blocked. However, they are uncomfortable. In children, enteral feeding is a complex procedure and can lead to developmental delay (Huband and Trigg 2000), so special care is required when considering or allowing enteral feeding to be used.

Nasogastric (NG) tube feeding is common practice in nursing for all age groups. Thousands of tubes are inserted daily without incident, however, there is a small risk that the nasogastric tube can be misplaced into the lungs or moving out of the stomach, if correctly inserted into the stomach initially. The NPSA (2005) have produced an algorithm to help confirm the position of the nasogastric tube. Note, however, that this algorithm neither replaces clinical judgement nor supersedes local trust policy. A chest x-ray and testing of the aspirate with pH indicator paper will ensure the nasogastric tube is in the correct place and position.

The auscultation of air insufflated through the feeding tube ('whoosh test') (NPSA 2005a) and use of blue litmus paper to test the pH of the aspirate *should not* be used to confirm the position of the tube (NPSA 2005). It must be remembered that patients, especially the elderly or confused, may not want and refuse a nasogastric tube, and may repeatedly pull the tube out. It is important to ensure that the patient understands why the tube is required.

Box 8.3   Reasons for Insertion

Nasogastric tube (NG) feeding (for short term)
Percutaneous endoscopically placed gastrostomy (PEG) feeding (for long term feeding)
Nasoduodenal tubes
Nasojejunal tubes
Jejunostomy tubes
Dysphagia
Palliative care
Unconscious patient
Children with chronic conditions, e.g., cystic fibrosis, prolonged lack of eating can result in:

> Developmental delay, e.g., learning problems appropriate to social behaviour at meal times
> An obstruction of the oesophagus
> Loss of swallowing reflex
> Oesophageal fistula
> Unconscious patient
> Post-operative patient.

(Huband and Trigg 2000)

REFER TO PROCEDURE: INSERTION OF NASOGASTRIC TUBE

Principles of Nutritional Support

For short term use, a 12 french gauge (FG) small bore NG tube may be used for insertion into an adult patient. This kind of tube is more comfortable and easier to tolerate than wide bore NG tubes, which are used to empty the stomach contents post-operatively (e.g., after gastric surgery or bowel obstruction). The tube needs to be changed weekly (if not more frequently) and whenever it is blocked, obstructed or removed by the patient. An 8 FG is used for longer periods while a gastrostomy is used for permanent care. Enteral feeding can be administered intermittently or continuously via an administration set or controlled pump, or by bolus administration. It is a clean procedure and nurses should adhere to aseptic procedures when dealing with these modes of feeding.

Nasogastric feeding involves a number of processes. They include: explaining the procedure to the patient and obtaining consent; providing psychological reassurance regarding the need for such feeding and tube insertion; washing hands and wearing an apron; checking the patient's identity; and checking nose and face for soreness or pressure. Once inserted, check the tube for signs of displacement and that it is in the correct position according to trust policy and NPSA (2005) guidelines. Then prepare the prescribed feed and enteral administration set, and infuse the feed through the set to expel air. After connecting the administration set to the NG tube aseptically and commencing the feed, ensure the patient is comfortable and monitor the need for mouth care. Observe for nausea, dyspnoea or diarrhoea, 'flush' the NG tube on completion of the feed, record the volume of a fluid balance chart and change the administration set every 24 hours to minimise the risk of bacterial contamination and growth (NPSA 2005, Brooker and Waugh 2007).

Percutaneous endoscopically gastrostomy (PEG) feeding is recommended if the digestive system is still working well but nutritional support is required for more than a few weeks. A feeding tube is inserted surgically through an opening into the stomach, held by a stitch and a small inflated balloon under the skin or by flange around the tube under the skin.

LEARNING ACTIVITY 8.2

John is a 30 year old man with Down's Syndrome who has been admitted to hospital for investigations. The Speech and Language Therapist (SALT) wants to introduce PEG feeding because John at times finds it hard to swallow. However, John's elderly mother, who cares for him at home, is concerned that introducing a PEG feed may prove to be problematic without support. You share this concern.
  What is the most appropriate course of action?

Parenteral feeding is only used when enteral feeding is unsuitable, i.e., when the gastrointestinal (GI) tract is not functioning or cannot fully meet the nutritional needs of the patient. It is used for those who are unable to ingest, digest or absorb sufficient oral or enteral feeding. It may enable children with congenital and acquired conditions to survive (e.g., those who have had major bowel resection, extensive inflammatory disease of the GI tract). However, it is costly and the decision to use it should not be taken lightly. Feeding is administered via a central venous catheter or, for a short time, via a peripheral route and it requires multidisciplinary team collaboration between patient and carer, nurse, dietician, doctor, pharmacist, SALT and specialist nutritional nurse, among others.

Where enteral feeding occurs for more than one month, the gastrostomy tube may be replaced with a balloon made from silicone. The button is secured in place by a balloon or dome inside the stomach (Griffiths 1996). Being able to handle the tube requires an amount of manual dexterity from the patient so may not be suitable for some older patients (Thomas and Bishop 2007), those with arthritis or some weakness or paralysis of the hand.

REFER TO PROCEDURE: CARE OF PEG TUBE

The frequency of enteral feeding and amounts to be administered are usually prescribed by the medical team or dietician. The feed is prepared in accordance with the patient's needs. A standard formula includes protein, carbohydrate, fat, minerals and vitamins in specific proportions as prescribed by the medical team and dietician. The feed can then be administered intermittently, continuously or by bolus amounts. If administered intermittently, three to 500ml amounts are infused over 30 minutes. For continuous infusions this occurs over a 24 hour period via an infusion pump and at a continuous rate, while for bolus administration, a syringe is used to administer the feed into the stomach.

There are ethical concerns regarding the use of such invasive techniques in certain situations. These include discontinuing to feed or hydrate patients who refuse food or fluids as sips of water or ice cubes may be all the patient wants. There is insufficient evidence to justify refusing trialling tube-feeding patients with dementia and more research is required regarding alternative methods (Biernacki and Barratt 2001, Gillick 2000). For those with anorexia sectioned under the Mental Health Act (1983), enforced treatment as part of their overall treatment is legal.

Professional Responsibility Regarding Nutrition and Feeding

Nurses need to ensure that patients receive adequate nutrition when patients are unable to use their limbs, have lost coordination of their limbs, are partially sighted or blind, or have a mouth injury. Such nursing interventions are vital in helping patients maintain or improve their nutritional status. Through assessment and screening to provide an holistic approach regarding nutrition, nurses are able to recognise who is at risk of malnutrition, identify who is not eating, identify treatment (oral, enteral, parenteral support) required, and monitor and review nutritional support within a multidisciplinary team (MDT) approach, as supported by the Essence of Care document (NHS Modernisation Agency 2003, NICE 2006). By clearly identifying who is responsible for screening and ensuring all staff have access to and use screening assessment tools and equipment (e.g., weighing scales) (NICE 2006), patient nutritional requirements may usually be met.

Meeting patients' nutritional needs often requires involvement from the patient, family, carer, and MDT. It is important that the menu provides a choice so that patients can choose meals they will eat and which meet their dietary requirements.

It is important to promote a conducive environment for meals. This may involve providing a dining room or removing vomit bowls or commodes and shutting sluice doors during meal times. Washing hands before serving meals, taking patients to the toilet, emptying stoma and/or catheter bags before meals, positioning patients correctly to facilitate eating, providing utensils to facilitate eating for the older person to use (especially those who have had a stroke or have arthritis), serving food at the correct temperature and in an attractive fashion, explaining where and what the food is, especially to those with visual impairments – are all beneficial methods of ensuring that patients' nutritional needs are met. Providing alternatives if a meal is missed, fortification, smaller, frequent meals, using full fat milk, using full fat dairy products, high energy snacks between meals (biscuits, cakes), and maintaining hydration when people have an inadequate oral intake of fluids can also prove beneficial to ensure patients receive sufficient nutrients to meet their dietary needs, i.e., protein, carbohydrates, fats, vitamins.

Oral Hydration

Healthy individuals maintain their hydration levels by drinking fluids orally. This is a normal, non-invasive procedure that usually does not lead to complications. For those where this route is contraindicated (e.g., due to loss of swallowing reflex, vomiting, or unconsciousness) alternative approaches may be required. For instance, enteral fluids or subcutaneous (S/C) fluids may be used to provide and maintain hydration. Thus, a careful assessment is required. This requires an assessment of normal fluid intake and fluid preferences and of physical and psychosocial factors disrupting fluid intake. Assessment results must be documented, especially since daily fluid requirements vary from individual to individual.

Fluid Intake

Patients should be encouraged to drink between 1.5 and 3 litres in a 24 hour period, depending upon their condition and situation. However, infants and small children have little fluid reserve and so are at an increased risk of fluid and electrolyte imbalance with excess fluid intake. An older person requires a higher intake of fluid because the kidneys become less efficient in producing concentrated urine, are less sensitive to and responsive to the thirst sensation, and struggle to maintain body temperature and prevent **dehydration** in hot weather. Higher intake can be facilitated by sensitively and tactfully ensuring patients have a glass and jug of water within easy reach and ensuring they drink a glass of water regularly. A fluid balance chart should be used to monitor fluid intake and output. SALT and Occupational Therapy (OT) assessment may be used to promote safety and independence, while mouth and teeth care should be used to promote and encourage fluid intake and ensure that hydration and fluid intake is maintained.

LEARNING ACTIVITY 8.3

From your clinical area, e.g., adult, children, mental health, elderly, medically infirm, identify what items are used to ensure the patient drinks and how other drinks are offered.

- Is this sufficient to meet their homeostatic and hydrational needs?
- How does your clinical area ensure that a patient is drinking regularly?
- What drinks are offered?
- Is this sufficient?

Fluid Replacement Therapy

For those who are NBM (nil by mouth) intravenous fluids (I/V) or subcutaneous fluids (S/C) may be used to provide and maintain hydration, to maintain fluid, electrolyte and acid-base balance, to provide nutrients (e.g., TPN), to replace fluids and correct electrolyte imbalances and to administer drugs (e.g., chemotherapy). This is a short term method as in the long term it can block the peripheral vein. If it is subject to referral the medical team, a Speech And Language Therapist (SALT) and dietician may be required for fluid replacement. The fluids are administered directly into a vein as a means of volume replacement, restoring and maintaining fluid and electrolyte balance, for nutritional purposes or to administer drugs. Superior vena cava may be used for long term therapy, to dilute and prevent damage to the peripheral vein.

Subcutaneous infusions (S/C) or hypodermoclysis is used increasingly to provide treatment for mild to moderate dehydration, to provide fluid replacement and maintain hydration in older frailer patients, and as a form of palliative care (thereby avoiding the need for hospital-isation for rehydration). This method is suitable for any environment, is convenient and cost effective. Sites used include thighs, abdomen, chest wall and areas over the scapula. The selec-tion should be made after discussion with the patient and consideration of their comfort and skin condition. There is a risk of swelling, discomfort or inflammation locally, while fluid overload is unusual.

Fluids infused are classified as isotonic (used to restore blood volume), hypotonic (used to treat cellular dehydration and promote waste elimination by the kidneys) or hypertonic (drawing fluid out of the cells and into the interstitial compartments, the vascular compart-ment and to expand vascular volume). Hypertonic solutions such as saline solutions cause an increase in the heart rate and contractility and a reduction in peripheral vascular resistance (Protheroe and Nolan 2001).

Summary

The nurse's role in assessing, monitoring and providing for patients' nutritional and hydration needs is central. It ensures that individuals receive sufficient fluids and nutrients for their body's requirements; it prevents nutritional and fluid imbalance; and it promotes recovery from illness.

PROCEDURE: INSERTION OF NASOGASTRIC TUBE USING AN INTRODUCER

Before inserting a nasogastric tube check in the medical and nursing notes for potential complications, i.e., anatomical position of the nasal passages and oesophagus, obstructions (as they can prevent clear insertion of the nasogastric tube), resulting in pain, discomfort and further complications.

Action	Rationale
Explain and discuss the procedure to the patient and obtain consent	Ensures the patient understanding and consent gain is valid and informed
Sit the patient in the semi-upright position in bed or chair, supporting the head with pillows and closing the door/drawing the curtains	Allows the tube to be inserted easily and ensures epiglottis not obstructed by the oesophagus

Action	Rationale
	Maintains patient privacy, dignity and comfort
Agree upon a signal before the procedure the patient can use to communicate, if in difficulty	Allows the patient to have control over the procedure and is less frightened
Measure the distance on the tube from the patient earlobe to bridge of nose, allowing for distance from here to the bottom of the xiphisternum	Ensures appropriate length of tube is inserted into the stomach
Wash hands and assemble the equipment aseptically on a dressing trolley	Minimises cross-infection
Check the patient's nostrils by asking them to sniff with one nostril closed	Identifies any obstructions liable to prevent insertion of the tube
Follow the manufacturer's instructions regarding preparing nasogastric tube, e.g., inject sterile water for injection into the tube and lubricate proximal end of the tube with lubricating jelly	Water activates and coats the inside of the tube and on the tip, lubricating tube facilitates the insertion of the tube, allowing easy withdrawal of the introducer
Insert the rounded end of the tube into the clear nostril, slide backwards and inwards along the nose to the nasopharynx Withdraw if an obstruction is felt and try again in a slightly different direction, or the other nostril	Facilitates the passage along the natural anatomy of the nose
Ask the patient to mouth-breathe, sip some water and swallow as the tube passes down the nasopharynx, unless swallowing is contraindicated	Redirects the patient's attention elsewhere Swallowing closes the glottis and enables the tube to pass into the oesophagus
Advance the tube through the pharynx as the patient swallows and until the predetermined mark has been reached. If the patient is in distress remove the tube immediately	Tube may accidentally be inserted into the trachea Distress may indicate tube is in the bronchus
Remove the introducer by using gentle traction. If difficult to remove, remove the nasogastric tube as well	Introducer sticking in the tube may indicate the tube is in the bronchus
Secure the tube securely with tape to the nose	Holds the tube in place Ensures comfort

(Cont'd)

Action	Rationale
Measure the visible part of the tube from the tip of the nose and record in the care plan Mark the tube at the exit site	Recording assists in detecting movement of the tube
Check the position of the tube to confirm it is in the stomach by, i x-ray chest and upper abdomen ii aspirating 2 mls of stomach content and testing with pH indicator strip: pH 5.5 indicates gastric acid; if pH 6.0 or above *do not* commence feed. X-ray or reposition tube iii wait for 1 hour before commencing feed iv flush with 20 mls or air to clear other substances	Ensures feeding can begin X-ray is the most accurate method of confirmation for those with altered anatomy, those aspirating or unconscious with no gag reflex Indicates if contents are gastric acid or bronchial secretions Increases risk of tube being incorrectly placed May raise pH of stomach
Do not ascultate (introduce air and check for bubbling). Use litmus paper or note for absence of respiratory distress	Ascultation is an inaccurate or unreliable method of checking as it can result in false results
Ensure patient is comfortable before removing and disposing of equipment as per trust policy	In case the tube requires reinserting or repositioning
Remove gloves and apron and wash hands as per trust policy	Minimises cross-infection
Document tube insertion, any abnormal findings or difficulties with the insertion	Communicates care

PROCEDURE: INSERTION OF NASOGASTRIC TUBE WITHOUT USING AN INTRODUCER, E.G., RYLE'S TUBE

A ryle's tube is used for drainage of the stomach contents whereas a fine bore tube is used for feeding.

Action	Rationale
Follow the first six steps as for 'Insertion of Nasogastric Tube Using an Introducer'	Follow the first six steps as for 'Insertion of Nasogastric Tube Using an Introducer'
Lubricate 15–20 cms of the tube with a thin layer of lubricating jelly	Reduces the friction between the mucous membrane and the tube

Action	Rationale
Insert the proximal end of the tube into the clear nostril and slide backwards/inwards along the floor of the nostril to the nasopharynx. If obstructed, withdraw the tube and try again in a slightly different direction or the other nostril	Facilitates the passage of the tube following the natural anatomy of the nose
As the tube passes down the nasopharynx ask the patient to sip some water and then swallow	Redirects the patient's attention elsewhere Swallowing closes the glottis and enables the tube to pass into the oesophagus
Advance the tube through the pharynx as the patient swallows until the tape marked on the tube is reached If the patient is in distress, remove the tube	Distress may indicate the tube is in the bronchus
Secure the tube on the nose with tape	Holds the tube in place and ensures comfort
Check the tube is in position by, i x-ray of the chest and upper abdomen ii aspirating 2 mls of stomach contents after 1 hour. Before aspirating flush the tube with 20 mls of air clear of any other substances iii pH 5.5 indicates tube is in the stomach iv pH 6.0 or above indicates the tube is in the wrong place so reposition and x-ray	X-ray is the most accurate method of confirmation in those with altered anatomy; those aspirating or unconscious with no gag reflex Leave for 1 hour as a raise in pH may indicate an inaccurate result The pH indicates tube may be in the wrong place
Do not auscultate (introduce air and checking for bubbles). Use litmus paper and note if the patient is in respiratory distress	Auscultation is an inaccurate or unreliable method resulting in false results being produced
Follow last three steps as for 'Insertion of Nasogastric Tube Using an Introducer'	Follow last three steps for 'Insertion of Nasogastric Tube Using an Introducer'

PROCEDURE: CARE OF PERCUTANEOUS ENDOSCOPICALLY PLACED GASTROSTOMY (PEG) TUBE

This should be done daily and begins 36–48 hours following insertion. It helps maintain skin integrity and detect any problems, e.g., infection, skin breakdown.

Action	Rationale
Explain and discuss the procedure with the patient and obtain their consent	Ensures patient understanding and consent is informed and valid

(Cont'd)

Action	Rationale
Perform the procedure aseptically while also showing patient social cleaning technique, i.e., using soap and water around the site	Minimises cross-infection which can also be reduced greatly if the patient is self caring for the site
Remove the dressing if in place Observe the peristomal skin and stoma site infection, irritation and excoriation	Gains access to the stoma site Detects complications and instigates appropriate treatment
Note number of measuring guide on tube closest to the end of the external fixation device and ease fixation device away from the abdomen	Ensures the gastrostomy tube is reattached to the fixation device in the correct position
Clean the site with sterile solution and dry thoroughly	Removes exudates, prevents infection and skin excoriation
Rotate the tube 360 degrees	Prevents the tube adhering to the sides of the stoma tract
Gently push the external fixation device against the abdomen	Enables the tube to reattach to the fixation device
Gently pull the tube and attach the fixation device	Ensures the tube is correctly secured
Ensure the correct point on the measuring device on the tube is placed closest to the end of the fixation device	Ensures the tube is correctly secured If the patient gains weight release the external fixation device slightly to prevent **necrosis** of the stoma site
Don't cover the site with a new dressing unless discharge or leakage noted from the site	Encourages wound healing
Don't use bulky dressings under the external fixation device	Can increase the pressure on the internal retention disc or retention balloon and increase risk of tissue necrosis and ulceration of the stomach
Advise the patient not to use talcum powder or moisturising cream around the site	Prevents infection and/or skin irritation Grease on the skin can cause the external retention device to slip, allows movement of the tube and increases the risk of leakage and infection Creams and talcum powder can affect the tube material causing it to leak or stretch

PROCEDURE: CARE OF INFUSIONS

Action	Rationale
Explain and discuss the procedure with the patient and obtain consent	Ensures patient understanding and consent is informed and valid
Use non-dominant hand/arm considering patient/client wishes	Maximises independence and minimises inconvenience
Support the hand/arm with a pillow or lightly bandage with a splint as per trust policy	Muslims use left hand for personal cleansing and right hand for feeding Ensures safety and comfort Splint immobilises arm if patient/child at risk of becoming confused or restless
Secure cannula site with sterile dressing Record date of insertion and type of administration set used Change cannula site every 72 hours in accordance with manufacturer's/trust instructions Use aseptic procedure and standard precautions at all stages	For security purposes and reduces incidence of infection Prevents contaminants/micro-organisms entering the cannula site Protects staff from potential infection
IV bags of fluid should be changed using aseptic technique Change administration set every 72 hours as per manufacturer and trust policy document	Prevent contaminants/micro organisms entering the set Reduces the risk of infection
Check cannula site for signs of infection, e.g., redness, swelling, pain Check dressing around cannula and change aseptically if loose, wet, blood stained If dressing is intact, dry and clean, leave until cannula requires resiting or removing	Indicates phlebitis, infection or another complication Prevents cross-infection

FEEDING A PATIENT

Positioning

Sit down in a position of comfort and at same eye contact as the patient
Place the table at a suitable height and within reach for the patient
Consider the patient's position and comfort
Place where the patient can see the food
Method of feeding should be as normal as possible
Where feeding required, it enables the nurse to monitor amounts eaten and whether further assessment/support required
Encouragement and motivation maintains dignity and independence.

Diet Choice

Appearance
Taste
Temperature
Consistency
Supplements
Choice from the menu
Assist where required
Explanations, e.g., vegetarian, partially sighted
Smaller, individual meals
Finger foods for children, older people.

Utensils

Normal/adapted cutlery
Cut up food to manageable portions
Do not use spoons for everything; use a knife and fork where possible
Do not use bibs (dignity)
Use napkins instead.

Timing/Place

Remove equipment, e.g., urinals, commodes, vomit bowls
Adopt a quiet, relaxed atmosphere
Consider use of a separate dining room
Wash hands before and after meals
Toileting before and after meals.

Documentation

Nursing notes
Diet sheets
Fluid balance charts
Swallowing assessments by SALT.

(Weetch 2001)

References

BAPEN (2003) *The Malnutrition Universal Screening Tool (MUST)*. BAPEN, Maidenhead.

Biernacki, C and Barratt, J (2001) Improving the Nutritional Status of Patients with Dementia, *British Journal of Nursing* 10(17): 1105–1114.

Bond, S (1997) *Eating Matters: A Resource for Improving Dietary Care in Hospitals*, Newcastle upon Tyne, Centre for Health Services Research Newcastle.

Brooker, C and Waugh, A (eds) (2007) *Foundations of Nursing Practice. Fundamentals of Holistic Care.* Mosby, Edinburgh.

Brozek, J (1990) Effects of Generalised Malnutrition on Personality, *Nutrition* 6: 389–395.

Chandra, RK (1990) The Relation Between Immunology and Disease in Elderly People, *Ageing* 19: S25–S31.

Collier, J (2002) Using a Nutritional Assessment Tool in the Hospital Setting, *Nurse2Nurse* 2(6): 32–33.

DH (2001) *Essence of Care*. DH, London.

Devlin, M (2000) The Nutritional Needs of the Older Person, *Professional Nurse* 16(3): 951–965.

Dougherty, L and Lister, S (2006) *Royal Marsden Hospital Manual Procedures*. Blackwell Publishing, Oxford.

Gillick, MR (2000) Rethinking the Role of Tube Feeding in Patients with Advanced Dementia, *New England Journal of Medicine* 342: 206–210.

Green, SM and Watson, R (2005) Nutritional Screening and Assessment Tools for Use by Nurses: Literature Review, *Journal of Advanced Nursing* 50(1): 69–83.

Griffiths, M (1996) Single-Stage Percutaneous Gastrostomy Button Insertion: A Leap Forward, *Journal of Parent Enteral Nutrition* 20(3): 237–239.

Huband, S and Trigg, E (2000) *Practices in Children's Nursing*. Churchill Livingstone, Edinburgh.

Huddleston, KC et al. (1993) Nutritional Support of the Critically Ill Child, *Critical Care Nursing Clinics of North America* 5(1): 65–78.

Ledsham, J and Gough, A (2000) Screening and Monitoring Patients for Malnutrition, *Professional Nurse* 15(11): 695–698.

Lennard-Jones, J (1992) *A Positive Approach to Nutrition as Treatment*. Kings Centre, London.

Malik, M et al. (2004) *Nursing Knowledge and Practice. Foundations for Decision Making,* 2nd edn. Baillere Tindall, Edinburgh.

Marik, PE et al. (2001) Early Enteral Nutrition in Acutely Ill Patients: A Systematic Review, *Critical Care Medicine* 29: 2264–2270.

Mental Heath Act (1983) HMSO, London.

NHS Modernisation Agency (2003) *Essence of Care: Patient-Focussed Benchmarks for Clinical Governance.* www.modern.nhs.uk/home/key/docs

National Collaborating Centre for Acute Care (2006) *Nutrition Support in Adults: Oral Nutrition Support, Enteral Tube Feeding and Parenteral Nutrition.* NCCAC, London. www.rcseng.ac.uk/ publications/docs/nutrition_support.guidelines

NPSA (2005) Reducing the Harm Caused by Misplaced Feeding Tubes. www.npsa.nhs.uk.advice

NPSA (2005a) *How to Confirm the Correct Position of Nasogastric Tubes in Infants, Children and Adults*. NPSA, London.

NICE (2006) *Nutritional Support in Adults, Clinical Guidelines 32*. NICE, London.

NMC (2007) *Guidance for the Introduction of the Essential Skills Clusters for Pre-Registration Nursing Programmes*. NMC, London.

Payne-James, J et al. (2001) *Enteral Nutrition: Tubes and Techniques of Delivery*. In Payne-James et al. (eds) *Artificial Nutritional Support in Clinical Practice,* 2nd edn. Greenwich Medical Media, London.

Protheroe, R and Nolan, J (2001) Which Fluid to Give? *Trauma* 3: 151–160.

Robinson, G et al. (1987) Impact of Nutritional Status on DRG Length of Stay, *Journal of Parenteral Nutrition* 11(1): 49–51.

Stratton, RJ et al. (2004) Malnutrition in Hospital Outpatients and Inpatients: Prevalence Concurrent Validity and Ease of Malnutrition Universal Screening Tool (MUST) for Adults, *British Journal of Nutrition* 92(5): 799–808.

Sullivan, DH (1992) Risk Factors for Early Hospital Readmission in a Select Population of Geriatric Rehabilitation Patients: The Significance of Nutritional Status, *Journal of American Geriatrics Society* 792–798.

Thomas, B (2001) *Manual of Dietetic Practice*. Blackwell Science, Oxford.

Thomas, B and Bishop, J (2007) *Manual of Dietetic Practice,* 4th edn. Blackwell Publishing, Oxford.

Weetch, R (2001) Feeding Problems in Elderly Patients? *Nursing Times Plus* 97(16): 60–61.

Windsor, JA et al. (1988) Wound Healing Response in Surgical Patients: Recent Food Intake is More Important than Nutritional Status, *British Journal of Surgery* 75: 135–137.

Zainal, G (1994) Nutritional Demands, *Nursing Times* 20(91): 38, 57–59.

9

Elimination

Learning Outcomes

This chapter is designed to help you:

o   understand the functioning of the bowel and urinary system
o   identify common problems associated with urination and defaecation
o   identify the complications associated with bowel and urinary disorders
o   understand the interventions associated with these problems
o   learn the principles of catheter care
o   recognise the professional role of the nurse when providing care for individuals with elimination difficulties.

Introduction

Continence, bladder and bowel care form an important part of nursing. They are among the subjects covered in the Essence of Care document (DH 2001). Making a Difference (DH 1999) saw continence as a fundamental aspect of care, but found that care provision often falls below acceptable standards. According to the NMC (2007: 9), students need to be able to 'where relevant, apply knowledge of age and condition related anatomy and physiology when interacting with patients/clients'. Such fundamental considerations apply as much to continence, bladder and bowel care as to other areas.

Functions of the Urinary System

The urinary system plays an integral part in maintaining homeostatic balance in the body, ensuring unwanted waste products are excreted, water balance is maintained and blood pressure controlled. The urinary system includes two kidneys, two ureters, the bladder and urethra. Urine is formed when blood is filtered through the kidneys.

During the formative years of life the nerve supply to the bladder becomes complete and the toddler learns that the sensation in the bladder indicates a need to urinate. This process is facilitated when the nerve fibres in the bladder wall stretch and impulses pass to the spinal cord, initiating spinal reflex and causing detrusor muscle contraction, internal sphincter relaxation and urination.

When such anatomical developments are complete, the urethral sphincters and bladder are controlled by a more complex nervous system. Nerve impulses from the spinal cord pass to the cerebral cortex of the brain where the impulses are interpreted and the need to urinate is determined. The cerebral cortex then sends nerve impulses back to the spinal cord, bladder and internal sphincter. The detrusor muscle contracts, causing a reflex relaxation of internal sphincter and voluntary relaxation of the external sphincter, allowing urine to pass along the urethra. Once the bladder is empty, the nerve impulses cease, the detrusor muscle stops contracting and the sphincter closes. This process is aided by an increase in the pelvic pressure, **aldosterone** and **anti-diuretic hormone** (ADH), which maintain fluid and electrolyte homeostasis by increasing the permeability of the renal tubules and water.

Where a patient does suffer from elimination problems, nurses need to identify the patient's 'normal' elimination patterns, including a consideration of how frequently they usually urinate or defecate. The nurse needs to identify how mobile and dextrous the patient is (can they mobilise out to the toilet? Can they unzip their clothing?). The assessment also needs to take account of any known medical conditions (e.g., Crohns disease), whether any factors (certain foods, for example) are known to aggravate the problem and how the patient might be able to manage the problem (through use of laxatives or self-catheterisation, for example). Finally, the assessment needs to consider the home situation (for example, where the toilet is situated) and the patient's psychology (for example, states of anxiety or depression or a need for reassurance).

It is important to record any symptoms and duration of the problem(s). Assess and observe symptoms such as dribbling, dysuria, enuresis, frequency, hesitancy, incomplete emptying, poor urinary flow, retention, incontinence, colour, and consistency of stool. Ascertain if there is a stoma and consider measures that may be used to promote urination or defaecation.

Where long term incontinence is not managed or resolved by toileting (to promote muscle tone), increase fluid intake (to eliminate bacteria present) and hygiene care (of genitalia), consider the use of pads, sheaths or catheters (long term or intermittent) to maintain continence and prevent skin breakdown from constantly washing the patient. Also consider the potential role of education and lifestyle changes, and involving continence advisors, who may be able to provide alternative measures to promote continence.

Other factors to be aware of when promoting continence include the developmental stage of the patient (e.g., whether the patient is toilet trained), lack of privacy when using the commode; does the patient use pads; do they have any psychological issues (such as anxiety, stress due to lack of control, embarrassment), and any lack of suitable facilities, i.e., toilet. This may be hindered by immobility, dehydration, constipation, reduced fluid intake, diet that exacerbates the problem(s), disease or injury (cystitis, kidney failure, diabetes, stroke, dementia, head injury), neurological problems (resulting in frequency), gynaecological surgery, prostate surgery (resulting in reduced urinary output), medication, e.g., diuretics, opioids, antibiotics, and caffeine resulting in increased frequency.

Attempts need to be made to promote a return to 'normal' patterns of elimination. Treatment might include a number of aspects. It is likely to include encouraging a balanced, high fibre, diet and plenty of fluid intake (to promote normal bladder tone, homeostasis and elimination of micro-organisms that may be causing an infection). It is important where possible to ensure there are suitable facilities (for example, a toilet nearby), provide suitable aids (e.g., raised toilet seats, velcro fastenings instead of zips or buttons to facilitate easy removal of clothing when visiting the toilet), and promote mobility. It is necessary to review the patient's medication (for example, avoiding analgesics as they can result in constipation). Finally, consider the patient's cultural and religious needs. Throughout the process it is important to be aware of and control one's own attitude (avoiding demeaning comments and facial expressions that express disgust, for example).

Urinary Incontinence

Urinary incontinence affects all age groups. There are numerous types (stress, urge, overflow, reflex, functional). Each is likely to result in isolation, loneliness, low self esteem, shame, embarrassment and a disruption in the activities of living. The DH (2000) suggests that urinary incontinence occurs in one in five women and one in ten men over the age of 65, while 500,000 children experience bed wetting.

Incontinence is a treatable condition (DH 2000). Sufferers should feel confident about asking for assistance in order to promote continence. The patient may be placed near a toilet for regular two-hourly toileting (this promotes normal bladder tone and the patient controls when they wish to eliminate). The patient should avoid caffeine drinks and empty the bladder before bedtime (this minimises disturbing sleep patterns and urinating overnight).

Forms of care include provision of drinking fluids during the day (to eliminate any micro-organisms), pelvic floor exercises (to promote the tone of the pelvic floor), maintaining fluid balance charts (to monitor homeostasis), and referring to the continence nurse specialist as required.

Patients with poor manual dexterity may be unable to remove clothing with zips or buttons so velcro should be used, and wraparound skirts for women. Aids such as pads, sheaths and catheters should be used initially only if continence promotion has failed.

Catheters

Catheters are hollow tubes usually inserted via the urethra into the bladder. They serve many functions. They are used to empty the bladder, determine residual urine, irrigate the bladder, bypass an obstruction, relieve retention, introduce cytotoxic drugs, allow bladder functions to be performed, monitor acutely ill patients, relieve incontinence and avoid complications during the insertion of radioactive caesium. There are many problems associated with catheters. They can cause infection (as identified earlier), trauma and perforation. They also make an intimate activity public, resulting in self-consciousness.

Urinary catheterisation involves the insertion of a tube into the bladder using aseptic technique for the purpose of evacuating fluids (Dougherty and Lister 2006). This should only be used after alternative methods have been considered and the patient need for catheterisation has been assessed. The assessment should consider the clinical needs of the patient, anticipated duration of the catheterisation, patient preference and any risk of infection. NICE (2003) states that catheterisation should be reviewed regularly and catheters should be removed as soon as possible.

Tenke et al. (2004) estimates 15 to 25 per cent of patients admitted into hospital have a catheter inserted, while Winn (1996) estimated up to 45 per cent of all hospital infections are urinary tract infections (UTI). The incidence of infection is directly related to the duration of the catheter being in situ (Sedar and Mulholland 1999), with an average daily rate of 4 per cent in men and 10 per cent in women (Schaeffer 2002). Schaeffer (2002) also calculated the chance of remaining infection-free to be only 50 per cent. Acquiring a UTI prolongs hospitalisation, increases treatment costs and has negative psychological effects on the patient (for example, raising the fear of MRSA infection). The nurse should therefore make a priority of seeking to prevent the patient contracting a UTI.

Box 9.1   Catheters Used

Catheters Used

Intermittently
Short term (1–14 days)
Medium term (2–6 weeks)
Long term (up to 3 months)
Male catheters (40–44 cms)
    Lumen size 12–14 Charriere scale (Ch) or French Gauge (FG)
    18–30 Charriere scale or French Gauge for irrigation
    Balloon size 10–30 mls sterile water
Female catheters (23–26 cms)
    Lumen size 10–12 Charriere scale (Ch) or French Gauge (FG)
    Balloon size 10 mls sterile water
Children catheters (30 cms)
    Lumen size 6–10 Charriere scale (Ch) or French Gauge (FG)
    Balloon size 2.5–5 mls sterile water

(Pomfret 2000, Robinson 2001)

Under- or over-filling the balloon prevents drainage as the balloon sits over the catheter tip, causing pain, spasm, haematuria and bypassing, also putting pressure onto the bladder neck, resulting in necrosis and incontinence (Pomfret 2000, Robinson 2001). Controversy surrounds the use of anaesthetic gels due to assumptions (rather than empirical evidence) that catheterisations are painful for men but not for women (Tortora and Grabowski 2002). Where used, anaesthetic lubricating gel tends to be used for male catheterisation while for female catheterisation it is only used at the tip of the catheter, if used at all.

In the community clean, as opposed to sterile, intermittent catheterisation is accepted to be a safe, effective procedure with no increased risk of symptomatic urinary tract infection (Moore 1993). Intermittent self-catheterisation is used for those with multiple sclerosis, spina bifida or spinal injury, and those who are able to understand the process and have manual dexterity to self-catheterise, or who have a willing partner motivated to undertake the procedure. Intermittent catheterisation stops over-distension of the bladder, and prevents incontinence. It also enhances independence and self esteem as the patient decides when to catheterise themselves. However, improper techniques can increase the risk of urinary tract infections and failure to self-catheterise can cause tissue trauma and bacterial invasion (if the volume is greater than 500 millilitres) – hence the need to catheterise regularly.

The selection of the catheter type is based upon clinical need, patient preference and risk of infection. Reusable intermittent catheters are available as are hydrophilic catheters, which are associated with lower rates of infection. Lubrication is required where non-lubricated catheters are used. The manufacturer's instruction and the local trust's policy must be followed. NICE (2003a) guidelines recommend the following in relation to intermittent catheterisation – education and training, using a full aseptic technique, carrying out a risk assessment to determine whether asepsis is required, and ongoing training and support for patients and carers.

An advantage of intermittent catheterisation is that urinary tract infections are reduced, compared to the situation with an indwelling catheter, while the ability to maintain sexual activity is maintained (Naish 2003). How often an individual self-catheterises will vary, but one should seek to ensure that the bladder does not hold more than 500 millilitres of urine. More than this can cause nerve damage by overstretching the bladder (Barton 2000).

Suprapubic catheters are inserted through the anterior abdominal wall into the dome of the bladder under general or local anaesthetic, using a percutaneous system (Kirkwood 1999). They may be used for those with an enlarged prostate gland or urethral stricture. They allow the urethra to remain intact, which allows normal micturition to occur post-operatively reduces pain and discomfort, and increases independence. Intercourse can occur with less impediment (Fillingham and Douglas 1997, Wilson 1998). The incidence of urinary tract infections is also reduced although encrustation still occurs in susceptible patients (Winn 1998, Simpson 2001). The care of such catheters requires an aseptic technique for dressing the site, while soap and water is sufficient for cleaning the catheter itself (Fillingham and Douglas 1997).

Principles of Catheterisation

Male catheterisation should not be undertaken by student nurses. Female catheterisation can be undertaken by student nurses but under the direct supervision of a qualified nurse. An explanation of the procedure and consent should be obtained, and the woman's privacy, dignity and respect should be maintained.

REFER TO PROCEDURE: FEMALE URINARY CATHETERISATION

Principles of Catheter Care

Catheter care is vital to maintaining high standards of personal hygiene in order to reduce the risk of infection ascending via the catheter. Any crusts or discharge must be removed from the catheter as they can harbour micro-organisms. With uncircumcised men retract the foreskin, remembering to return the foreskin back on completion of the provision of catheter care. If the patient requests a bath, disconnect and spigot the catheter, reconnecting it after the bath. Meanwhile, ensure that the drainage does not touch the floor at any time. Ensure a closed system is maintained, wearing gloves before handling catheters and wash hands after.

The meatus should be washed and the catheter site cleaned twice daily. If an infection is suspected, send a catheter specimen of urine (CSU), change the catheter according to the manufacturer instructions and clinical need and ensure the bag is below bladder level but not touching the floor. Empty the urine bag regularly and record all output on a fluid balance chart. Encourage an increase in fluid intake (to expel any micro-organisms present), while checking for signs of infection. Bladder washouts should only be performed if the catheter is bypassing. If a patient is discharged home with a catheter, a long term catheter or leg bag should be used. They must also be educated about hand washing, emptying or changing the bag and provided with contact numbers (GP, DN, incontinence nurse specialist) in case of emergencies. Sexual activity may be an embarrassing topic for discussion so may not be discussed when a catheter is first inserted. The subject should be discussed when the patient feels comfortable in doing so and may include their partner.

Complications of Catheterisation

Dunn et al. (2000) suggested that aseptic technique has not reduced the incidence of catheter-associated urinary tract infections (CAUTI), but good practice, guidance, using sterile equipment and the aseptic technique (Ward et al. 1997, Saint et al. 1999) can help. Dunn et al. (2000) also suggested that there was no advantage in using antiseptic preparations to clean the urethral meatus prior to catheterisation. Urethral trauma and discomfort are minimised by using appropriate sterile, single-use lubricant or anaesthetic gel, and by having healthcare practitioners who have been trained in the insertion of catheters.

Complications can arise with urinary catheterisation. These include infection (due to incorrect size, technique), pain (due to detrusor spasm causing irritation, urethral/external urethral meatus causing irritation), blockage (due to debris or obstruction or kinks in the catheter, bag being blocked), urethral stricture, urethral trauma (due to the bag not being secured, damage to the bladder, urethra, external urethral meatus) and encrustations.

Urinary tract infections (UTIs) occur frequently with catheters (Penfold 1999, Pratt et al. 2001) because the urethra has been bypassed. Davenport and Keeley (2005) and DH (2004) both suggest that silver alloy-coated catheters could reduce catheter associated UTI (CAUTI) by up to 45 per cent by reducing bacterial adhesion on the catheter. DH (2004) concluded that further research was required to audit the cost implications. CAUTIs can also be prevented by ensuring the catheter is cleaned twice daily with warm soapy water as it prevents encrustation around the meatus occurring and removes the potential source of infection.

Drainage bags used should consist of a 'closed system' to reduce the incidence of infection. Each time the bag is drained the potential risk of an infection increases, so emptying the bag should be kept to a minimum. The drainage bag should be kept on a stand to ensure that the tap and bag do not touch the floor, with the bag kept below the bladder to prevent urine tracking back into the bladder and causing an infection. Above all, always use aseptic technique when inserting and/or dealing with the catheter (Pratt et al. 2001).

The bag should be changed according to clinical need, in the event of leaking, and according to manufacturer's instructions (Wilson 1998, Pratt et al. 2001) and local trust policy. If a leg bag is worn, it must be secured with velcro tape or leg straps as dragging on the catheter can cause an injury to the urethra and external urethral opening. If secured properly, leg bags can facilitate mobility, dignity and independence.

Bowel Care

Bowel care is a sensitive issue and providing effective care and management for problems associated with it can be problematic. Cadd et al. (2000) note that many patients are too embarrassed to discuss bowel function and delay reporting problems (such as blood in faecal matter). The nurse's role is to assess the cause of the problem, find solutions and provide holistic assessment, health education and health promotion, and ensure that the patient has coping strategies. This requires a sensitive and skilled approach drawing on both the nurse's communication skills and his or her understanding of elimination difficulties (Smith 2001).

Pathophysiology of Bowel Movement

Digestion and absorption occurs in the small intestine (duodenum, jejunum, ileum), where movement of the contents in the small intestine occurs by segmentation and peristalsis. Segmentation is the localised contraction of the intestine, where intestinal contents are mixed together and food particles are brought into contact with the mucosa for absorption. The contents remain here in the small intestine for three to four hours while the nutrients, electrolytes and water are absorbed. Action is controlled by the autonomic nervous system (Tortora and Grabowski 2002).

Faecal matter moves through the colon by peristalstic action, beginning in the middle of the transverse colon and quickly moves to the rectum. This is otherwise known as gastrocolic reflex (Tortora and Grabowski 2002). Faeces remain in the sigmoid colon until the need to defecate is stimulated. If this does not occur for hours, it results in constipation, which can be exacerbated by dehydration and lack of fibre. When stimulated, the faeces move into the rectum in preparation for defecation. The diaphragm, abdomen and levator muscles contract and the glottis closes. Peristaltic waves occur in the distal colon, the anal sphincter relaxes and the faeces are expelled (Tortora and Grabowski 2002).

This whole process develops during the formative years of life along with physical, psychosocial and motor development. Toddlers are unable to control their ability of where and when to defecate. Control is practised by potty training, and using the toilet instead of wearing nappies. A reduction in muscle strength, mobility and age can affect the defaecation process as the external sphincter may weaken, causing a reduction in sensation which can result in faecal soiling. Adults are often reluctant to seek help: they feel embarrassed over loss of independence and a return to child-like behaviour. Medication can also cause difficulties. For example, non-steroidal anti-inflammatory drugs (NSAIDs) cause diarrhoea, while analgesics can cause constipation.

Constipation

There is no accepted definition of constipation, as it depends upon individual interpretation. Walsh (1997) viewed constipation as 'delayed movement of the intestinal content through the bowel', characterised by infrequent, hard, dry stools that may be difficult to pass (Norton 1996, Winney 1998). A useful definition may be 'an alteration in normal bowel movements, resulting in the less frequent and uncomfortable passage of hard stools' (Walker 2007). Constipation may be secondary to bowel disease. A thorough assessment is required to ascertain the underlying cause of the constipation.

Kyle et al. (2005) developed a constipation risk assessment tool called the Eton Scale. This indicates key risk factors to be considered when assessing patients, while also providing advice and suggesting actions according to the patient's level of risk. When assessing patients without using this tool, consider changes that may have occurred in the patient's diet or fluid intake, how mobile they are, any medication taken, any changes in their normal routines and psychological status (Thompson et al. 2003, Kyle et al. 2005), bowel activity, volume, consistency and colour of the stool passed, presence of mucous, blood, undigested food or offensive odour and any pain or discomfort on defaecating (Peate 2003, RCN 2006). In doing so, valuable information of any potential underlying medical problem may be collected.

Constipation can also be affected by a lack of fibre, reduced intake of fluid, fruit and vegetables, a lack of exercise, medication, change in the environment, resulting in bulk and the reduction in mobility of the faecal matter along the colon. This can cause a number of problems. They include abdominal colic, pain, cramps, flatulence, bloating, lethargy, fatigue, feeling generally unwell, excessive straining, headache, nausea, increased confusion and changes in behaviour (e.g., irritability).

Management of Constipation

Constipation can be managed through encouraging a high fibre diet, increased fluid intake and exercise. Fluid intake and exercise adds moisture to faecal matter, which increases mobility through the colon, thus preventing constipation occuring. Medication should also be reviewed (e.g., some analgesics can cause constipation).

The management of constipation can be enhanced by administering an enema or suppository. Osmotic laxatives are not recommended either as the first line of use or for continued use as they can result in dehydration, due to watery stools being produced. Enemas are useful for impacted stools, while arachis oil enemas may be used when stools are hard and impacted. However, the type of laxative prescribed is dependent upon bowel frequency and stool consistency.

REFER TO PROCEDURE: ADMINISTRATION OF ENEMAS

REFER TO PROCEDURE: ADMINISTRATION OF SUPPOSITARIES

Diarrhoea

King (2002) viewed diarrhoea as an abnormal faecal discharge, usually characterised by the frequency at which it occurs and its watery appearance (e.g., a loose watery stool). It can be acute or chronic, secretory, osmotic or mixed. It may be due to the side effects of treatment (e.g., cancer treatment), medication (e.g., antibiotics), enteral feeding, infections (food poisoning, gastroenteritis), food intolerance, stress and anxiety, change in diet, allergy, travel, bowel disease (e.g., Crohn's disease, Ulcerative Colitis) or malabsorption (e.g., Coeliac).

Possible problems caused by diarrhoea include a loss in fluid, electrolyte and nutrient imbalance, dehydration, perianal soreness, flatulence, abdominal cramps and pain, nausea and vomiting, poor appetite, foul smelling stools, embarrassment, urgency and faecal soiling. No matter the underlying cause of diarrhoea it has physiological and psychological effects on the patient (e.g., embarrassment, loss of control). Coping mechanisms are required to help the patient deal with the problem, e.g., changing their diet, sleep changes, isolation and depression (Hogan 1998, Kornblau et al. 2000).

Such approaches need to be incorporated into nursing practice so that the cause of diarrhoea is established through assessment. Lack of a systematic assessment and poor documentation can result in poorly managed diarrhoea (Cadd et al. 2001, Smith 2001) A comprehensive assessment is essential and should include a consideration of history of onset, frequency and duration, consistency, the colour and form of the stool (including any presence of blood, fat or mucous), pain, weight loss, recent lifestyle changes, medication, dietary and fluid changes, or psychological issues of concern (Kornblau et al. 2000, King 2002, Chelvanayagam and Norton 2004). The episodes of diarrhoea need to be recorded on a stool chart. The nurse should encourage the patient to take frequent sips of water to replace lost water and electrolytes. Antidiarrhoeal drugs (e.g., loperamide) may be prescribed. The patient must have easy access to a bedpan, commode, or toilet, along with toilet paper. It is important to maintain the patient's privacy and dignity. Ventilation and air freshener can help to minimise embarrassment. It is helpful to assist the patient with perianal hygiene and to provide creams (to prevent skin damage) and clean clothing. Be sure to use a stool and fluid balance chart and adhere to infection control measures (e.g., use of hand washing, gloves and aprons, side room). Send a stool sample for microbial examination to ascertain the cause and subsequent treatment required. Provide the patient with psychological support 'to maximise comfort and dignity, deliver care with dignity, take a person centred care approach' (NMC 2007).

Faecal Incontinence

The Royal College of Physicians (1995) described faecal incontinence as the inappropriate or involuntary passage of faeces, often characterised by faecal soiling, the involuntary passage of faeces in a socially inappropriate place, the lack of awareness of the urge to defecate or confusing the sense to defecate with that of flatus. Individuals with long term physical disabilities, neurological conditions and learning disabilities are more likely to encounter problems with faecal incontinence. DH (2000) estimates that 1 per cent of adults at home and 17 per cent of very elderly people report symptoms of faecal incontinence.

Faecal incontinence is common in older people, with 15 per cent in the community over the age of 65 years being affected (Royal College of Physicians 1995). More women than men are affected. Faecal incontinence is underreported because of the nature of the condition: it is considered a 'taboo subject', socially stigmatised or repugnant, and as a result patients are often reluctant to speak about or seek help for such topics.

Children may suffer from a condition called **encopresis** (repeated involuntary faecal soiling of clothing by a child over four years of age). It is often confused with other childhood problems, e.g., fear of using the toilet. Approximately 1.5 per cent of children lack bowel control at their seventh birthday (Royal College of Physicians 1995). Heins and Ritchie (1985) describe encopresis as having a lack of bowel control and indicate that it is a symptom of an emotional disorder. They found that encopresis is associated with long term constipation and faecal impaction, where the receptors in the rectum are stretched and continually stimulated because the rectum is full of faeces. This results in a loss of signal and normal response to muscle contraction; hence encopresis. It can take up to six months for an overstretched rectum to return to normal functioning (Heins and Ritchie 1985).

Children suffering from encopresis may lack privacy for washing or changing. They may be seen as 'smelly' and be the focus of teasing and/or bullying by other children. They therefore tend to avoid participating in games at school, or undressing in public, for fear of embarrassment. It is important that a multidisciplinary approach is adopted to prevent further embarrassment, isolation, rejection and lowered self esteem. Involve the family or carer, friends, school, GP, incontinence nurse, Health Visitor and school nurse. Strategies such as providing education regarding diet and exercise, encouraging regular toileting (to regain control and response to the stretch receptor signals, contraction and relaxation of faeces being expelled) and providing children with private changing facilities when participating in group activities such as games are required. Ensure that the school is aware of the child's need to use the toilet frequently, the disruption this may cause and the need for psychological support.

The causes of faecal incontinence are numerous and include constipation, diarrhoea (due to irritable bowel disease), pelvic floor problems (loss of sensation, weak muscles or rectal prolapse), loss of sensation in the anal area (due to spina bifida, MS, stroke), sphincter abnormalities (after rectal surgery), dementia, lack of or poor access to toilet facilities, immobility, poor manual dexterity or medication.

Managing Continence Care

Bowel difficulties can cause a number of problems – embarrassment, low self esteem, urgency to defecate, perianal soreness, risk of pressure sores, patients hiding their clothing, financial difficulties (because of the cost of clothing, pads, laundry) and social problems (isolation and loneliness). Managing these problems requires sensitivity. It is important to identify the underlying cause in order to manage the problem. The NHS Modernisation Agency (2003) stated a need for an integrated continence service that spans both primary and secondary care settings by focusing upon healthy living. It indicated the need to provide specialist continence advice for maintaining faecal and urinary continence, and care if continence is lost. The underlying philosophy is that promoting continence will reduce the incidence of incontinence.

If a bowel problem is due to constipation, it may be treated by increasing fibre and fluid intake, placing the patient near the toilet, toileting regularly (to facilitate peristaltic control of the bowel wall) and involving the continence advisor for care and education. If the cause is impaired sensation or sphincter control (as with patients with multiple sclerosis (MS)), then administer enemas or suppositories. NICE (2003) provides guidance for those with chronic conditions. It recommends assessment and routine use of enemas or suppositories.

Anti-diarrhoeal drugs may be used if faecal incontinence is due to a very liquid stool (bulk-forming drugs are taken with fluid to increase stool size so people with a reduced fluid intake, such as patients with renal failure, may not benefit from taking these drugs. People with neuropathic damage may also not benefit from taking bulking agents as it is difficult to expel large stool mass). In extreme situations, surgery may be considered. For those patients with spinal injuries or dementia planned care is required.

Where continence is not achieved, assessment and re-assessment is required. Continue to encourage a high fibre diet, review the medication causing the diarrhoea or constipation and administer pain relief. Place the patient near the toilet to maintain privacy and dignity and ensure he or she is wearing suitable underwear and pads. Protective equipment may be used for beds and chairs. Provide skin care and barrier creams. It is important to adopt a multidisciplinary team approach and maintain professionalism (for example, not making demeaning comments or facial expressions).

DH (2000) states that no products should be used without an assessment of the patient's physical and cognitive capabilities and cause of the incontinence. Quality *not* quantity care is central to treatment *not* the cost of treatment, the use of performance indicators and audits to monitor progress. This ensures quality of service nationally for those with elimination difficulties.

Stoma Care

A stoma is a surgically created opening of the bowel or urinary tract to the abdominal wall as a diversionary procedure because either the colonic or urinary tract beyond the position of the stoma is no longer viable (Dougherty and Lister 2008). A bag or pouch can then be connected to the stoma to collect the waste outside the body. Whether the stoma is temporary or permanent, and what the size and shape of the stoma is, will depend upon the type of surgery performed and how much of the bowel or urinary tract has been removed.

Box 9.2   Reasons for Stoma Formation

Inflammatory bowel disease, e.g., ulcerative colitis, Crohn's disease
Neoplasia
Diverticular disease
Cancer
Injury to the bowel
Trauma
Neurological damage
Congenital disease

(Taylor 2005, Dougherty and Lister 2008)

The names of surgical procedures that create a stoma end with '-ostomy'. There are various types of 'ostomies'. They include:

- colostomy (end or loop) – where there is an opening from the large intestine to the abdominal wall
- ileostomy (end or loop) – where there is an opening from the small intestine to the abdominal wall
- urostomy – where there is a connection between the urinary tract and abdominal wall resulting in a urinary conduit.

Sometimes it is possible to create an internal pouch for the waste: this is known as pouch surgery. It is a complex surgical procedure and usually available only in specialist hospitals.

A colostomy may be formed from any section of the large bowel (sigmoid, descending, transverse or ascending). The position will dictate the output and consistence of faecal matter. At the sigmoid colon, faecal matter will be semi formed or formed, while higher in the colon, the faecal matter is more liquid in consistency. An end colostomy is commonly performed to manage cancer of the lower rectum or anus or because of diverticular disease. A loop colostomy is traditionally created to defunction (bowel distal to the stoma being rested) (Taylor 2005) an inflamed sigmoid in diverticular disease or distal anastomosis (Nugent 1999).

An ileostomy is formed when a section of ileum (usually the last 20 centimetres) is brought to the abdominal wall and the contents can empty into a bag (Black 2000a). An end ileostomy is when the entire colon, rectum and anus have been removed. This is permanent and commonly occurs in severe ulcerative colitis, familial polyposis and some cases of colorectal cancer. It is less commonly performed and used when it cannot be fashioned safely in those who are obese or have an unfavourable mesenteric anatomy. It looks similar to a loop ileostomy. A loop ileostomy, however, is temporary and allows for the healing of an anastomosis lower down in the bowel, allows for the healing of an ileo-anal pouch or helps the healing of a diseased bowel (Taylor 2005). A loop ileostomy is easier to site, is less bulky and easier to surgically close (Fazio and Wu 1997).

A double barrel stoma is formed when the caecum is removed, and end ileostomy and mucus fistula sit beside each other. It looks almost identical to a loop ileostomy, but on closer examination two separate stomas may be seen.

Urostomies are formed when the bladder is removed or diseased. A section of ileum is isolated and anastomosis formed with its mesentery vessels and remaining ends of the ileum. The isolated section is mobilised, the proximal end closed and the ureters once resected attached to the bladder and implanted at this end. The distal end is brought to the surface of the abdominal wall and everted to form a spout (Black 2000b, Fillingham and Fell 2004). Urine produced will contain mucous from the bowel used in its construction (Taylor 2005).

The stoma is positioned away from the umbilicus, scars, costal margin or anterior superior iliac spine, to ensure compatibility with clothing worn, i.e., avoid the waistline or belt areas as clothing may put pressure on the stoma resulting in leaks or trauma (Dougherty and Lister 2008). The site should be marked before it is formed (but this may not be possible in emergencies, e.g., following a road traffic accident). A healthy stoma should be above skin level, red and moist (pallor indicating anaemia). There should not be separation between the skin and mucocutaneous site and should not exhibit any evidence of erythema, rash, ulceration or inflammation. When complications occur, they usually take the form of diarrhoea and/or constipation, necrosis, detachment, recession, stenosis, prolapse, ulceration, parastomal herniation or fistula formation skin excoriation (www.surgical-tutor.org.uk/specialities/general/stoma, www.student.bmj.com/issues).

There are two main types of stoma bags – single piece systems which stick straight onto the skin or two piece systems with a separate flange (base) that stick to the skin with a bag attached. This enables the bag to be changed without removing the flange. Some bags have a second opening at the bottom to facilitate opening, which is most useful immediately post operatively and also for patients who have had an ileostomy, and require the bag to be changed regularly. Closed bags are used when the faecal matter is formed and is usually changed daily or twice daily. Modern stoma bags are fitted with a carbon or charcoal flatus filter that neutralises any odours, allows gas to escape and prevents the bag ballooning or detaching.

There are several types of pouches that fit over the stoma by a hydrocolloid wafer or flange (Taylor 2000). The pouch may be opaque or clear and often has a soft backing to absorb perspiration. A filter is built in, containing charcoal to neutralise odours when flatus occurs (Dougherty and Lister 2008). Pouches are designed to fit discreetly under clothing, are easy to change, leak proof and odour tight. Deodorisers are available in the form of drops or powders and are applied to the pouch (to deodorise the contents, absorb or mask odours), while sprays are sprayed into the air before changing or emptying the pouch (Burch and Sica 2005). Any problems with odour or leakage can be investigated and resolved by using alternative appliances or accessories.

Solutions and skin barriers are available to clean the stoma and skin. This can be seen in the box below.

Box 9.3   Solutions and Skin Barriers Available

Solution/Skin Barrier	Purpose
Mild soap and water, or water only	Ensures all soap residues are removed as may interfere with pouch adhesion
Creams, e.g., Chiron barrier cream	Used on peristomal skin as any residual surface film of grease prevents the appliance to stick Used for sensitive skin
Protective films, e.g., Cavilon no string barrier film	Acts as film on skin to prevent irritation and protection Newer films don't contain alcohol so may be used on broken skin. Older films do contain alcohol so should not be used
Protective wafers	Hypoallergenic, designed to cover and protect skin and allows sore and broken skin to heal Useful where there are cases of skin reactions or allergies to adhesives or an appliance
Seals/washers, e.g., salts, cohesive seals	Protects skin around the stoma Useful in folds in skin
Pastes, e.g., soft, stomahesive paste	Fills crevices in the skin to provide a smooth surface for the appliance
Protective pastes, e.g., orabase paste	Protects raw areas Doesn't contain alcohol so doesn't cause irritation
Powders, e.g., orahesive powder	Protects sore or raw areas without hindering the adhesion of the appliance
Adhesive preparations, e.g., saltair solution	Used when appliance doesn't adhere well to the skin because of leakage or uneven site
Adhesive removers, e.g., appeal wipes and spray	Some contain alcohol so do not use on broken skin

Stoma baseplate securing tapes, e.g., hydroframe, secuplast	Used when adhering baseplate to the skin due to parastoma hernia, prolapsed stomas or stoam sited near bony prominence
Thickening agents, e.g., morform sachet, Gel-X capsules	Helps solidify loose stoma output and reduce pouch noise
Convex devices, e.g., adapt ring convex inserts, soft seal range of appliances	Used to retract stomas

www.hed2.bupa.co.uk   www.patient.co.uk   www.student.bmj.com

Professional Responsibilities of the Nurse

Caring for patients with elimination needs can be problematic. In Western society elimination is an intimate activity not always freely discussed, while in Eastern society, great importance is placed upon not using the right hand to clean the genitalia as it is used to feed oneself. Addressing elimination needs requires an holistic approach, including assessment and working with the patient, family and multidisciplinary team (MDT) to achieve independence and allow patients to regain 'normal' elimination patterns. This approach is supported by the NMC (2007: 4), who state that students be able to 'demonstrate knowledge of effective interprofessional working practices which respect and utilise the contributions of members of the health and social care team'. Referrals may therefore be required to a continence advisor who can provide psychological support as well as practical aids, to promote continence and help patients adjust to their condition.

Such approaches also allow the nurse to gain a better understanding of the patient, ensuring their needs are met and that the nurse knows how to manage their problem. Therefore, approach the patient with sensitivity and respect for their dignity and privacy considering their emotional and psychological response to the condition. This is because the nurse is not just proactive in providing an appropriate physiological and psychological intervention to help overcome elimination difficulties, but also involved in providing health education to the general public to dispel the negative and misguided attitudes surrounding elimination problems.

Summary

NHS Modernisation Agency (2003) specifies that 'patients have direct access to professionals who can meet their continence needs and their services are actively promoted'. With this provision, the care described above can be achieved.

The importance of promoting continence cannot be overstated as the nurse's role is central in ensuring patients receive sufficient assistance. This requires an holistic assessment to ensure healthcare professionals work together with patients and carers. Through assessment, care can be planned, implemented, evaluated and reviewed regularly, taking into account the patient's lifestyle, culture, beliefs and behaviour.

Education is a vital and important aspect of this process and care provision so help may be sought to resolve symptoms, or problems that may occur. Sensitivity, tact and diplomacy are required to achieve this as well as promoting privacy and dignity. This may be achieved through the nurse's use of communication and interpersonal skills, explaining procedures at every stage and in language understood by the patient and their family.

LEARNING ACTIVITY 9.1

Mr W, a 72 year old man with a distended bladder.

'I attended the A&E and after some hours waiting was put on the inevitable trolley where a catheter was inserted (not very painful, but rather uncomfortable) by one of the urology doctors. After four hours, a bed was found for me in a side room – what had I done to deserve this I thought? I had a television (which was useless) and a rather nice washroom. Tentatively, I settled myself into my little room when a terrible damp area appeared beneath me wetting the whole of the bed – something I hadn't done for years.'

'The Staff Nurse was called who was informed that nothing was draining into the bag under the bed, but everything was leaking into the bed. She said she would get a doctor to insert another catheter. A couple of hours later, who should come along but a young blond girl, no older than my daughter, but with a 'Doctor' badge on her white coat. She said, "Oh yes, the catheter is leaking. I'll get another one." Off she goes and returns with another catheter and proceeds to take out the leaking one and insert the new one. Apparently, at the time it was found that my prostate was so enlarged that the new catheter would not go past it. She said, "I'll go and get a thinner one". If the urine wouldn't drain out of the thicker one, how the heck was it going to drain from the thinner one? Ours is not to wonder why and then she said, "Don't go away, I'll be back". I wasn't going anywhere.'

'After fifteen minutes she returned with a much longer catheter and proceeded to insert it. At one time she said, "It will go in." After a push and a shove, she finally got it where she wanted it. Then everything started to flow as it should have done in the first place. Three of the under-bed bags were filled in no time and I lost half a stone in weight.'

- From the patient's perspective, how does the experience (i) look, (ii) feel, and (iii) sound?
- From your perspective, how does (i) the patient's experience look and (ii) how do his comments sound?
- How do you feel about this patient's experience?
- How would you have changed the patient's care?

PROCEDURE: FEMALE URINARY CATHETERISATION

Action	Rationale
Explain and discuss the procedure with the patient	Ensures patient understanding and consent is informed and valid
Ensure good lighting available	Facilitates catheterisation

Action	Rationale
Wash and dry hands thoroughly; clean trolley with alcohol-based preparation and place equipment required on bottom shelf of the trolley	Reduces the risk of infection Reserve the top shelf for a clean working area and catheterisation
Take trolley to patient bedside and draw curtains/close the door Prepare trolley as per 'Procedure: Aseptic Technique'	Minimises air bourne contamination and reduces risk of infection into urinary tract
Prepare patient i close door/draw curtains ii lie patient in supine position with knees bent, hips flexed and feet apart iii raise bed to acceptable height Remove bed clothing to expose genitalia while still maintaining patient privacy and dignity	Ensures patient privacy, dignity, comfort and allows air bourne organisms to settle Enables genitalia to be seen clearly and facilitates catheterisation Prevents stooping/bending over Protects bed clothing and creates sterile area Maintains privacy and dignity
Wash and dry hands thoroughly, wear gloves and apron	Reduces risk of cross-infection and creates a sterile field
Separate labia minora to see urethral meatus	Gains better access to urethral orifice and helps prevent labial contamination of the catheter
Clean around the urethral orifice with single downward stroke toward the anus	Reduces cross-infection
Insert lubricating jelly nozzle into the urethra, squeeze jelly into the urethra, remove nozzle and discard the tube Alternatively, use anaesthetic gel following same procedure. If used, follow manufacturer's instructions and lubricate catheter tip before insertion	Lubrication prevents trauma and minimises discomfort Anaesthetic gel prevents trauma, facilitates catheterisation and minimises discomfort
Place catheter into receiver and place receiver between legs	Acts as a temporary container for urine to drain into
Introduce lubricated tip of catheter into urethra in an upward and backward direction. Advance 5–6 cms and do not force its insertion	Adopts anatomical structure of the urinary tract Prevents trauma/damage to urethra
Remove catheter gently if urinary flow stops or advance another 6–8 cms	Prevents balloon becoming trapped in the urethra

(Cont'd)

Action	Rationale
Inflate balloon according to manufacturer's instructions, having ensured urine flowing into the receiver Withdraw slightly and connect to the drainage system Support the catheter with velcro strap provided or tape and stand. Ensure catheter is not taut when mobilising or catheter lumen not occluded by the strap/tape/clothing	Inadvertently inflecting the balloon in the urethra causes pain and trauma Maintains comfort Reduces the risk of trauma to urethral and bladder neck Tape may interact with catheter material
Ensure patient is comfortable, area is dry and place call bell nearby Draw back curtains/open door	If wet/moist infection and skin irritation may occur
Measure urine output	Raises awareness of bladder capacity Monitors urine output
Dispose of equipment in yellow plastic clinical waste bag as per trust policy	Prevents environmental contamination
Document procedure, i.e., date, time, catheter details, any difficulties faced, review date	Legal and effective communication Evaluation

PROCEDURE: EMPTYING CATHETER BAG

Action	Rationale
Explain and discuss with patient the procedure	Ensures patient understanding
Wash and dry hands thoroughly Wear gloves and apron	Reduces risk of cross-infection
Clean the outlet valve on the drainage bag with an alcohol swab and drain urine into a container, e.g., jug or urinal	Reduces the risk of cross-infection Emptying drainage bag and measuring volume
Close the outlet valve and clean again with a new alcohol swab	Reduces the risk of cross-infection
Cover container and dispose of urine as per trust policy	Reduces environmental contamination

Action	Rationale
Dispose of gloves and apron as per trust policy	Reduces risk of infection
Document amount of urine drained on fluid balance chart	Effective communication

PROCEDURE: REMOVAL OF URINARY CATHETER

Action	Rationale
Identify time to remove catheter, which is usually in the morning	Any retention can be dealt with during the day
Explain and discuss with the patient and inform them of any potential problems Obtain consent	Ensures patient understanding and consent obtained is informed and valid
Draw the curtains/close the door Position the patient for the removal of the catheter, i.e., lie them down, legs apart and cover their modesty	Maintains privacy and dignity Accesses catheter for its removal
Wearing gloves and apron, clean the meatus and catheter	Reduces the risk of infection
Release leg support and deflate the balloon	Eases removal of the catheter Ensures complete deflation of the balloon for removal of the catheter; minimises pain, discomfort and trauma
Ask patient to breathe gently and quickly and remove catheter telling patient what is occurring	Relaxes pelvic floor muscles thereby reducing pain and/or discomfort
Tidy away the equipment and ensure patient made comfortable Encourage them to drink 2–3 litres of water a day Ensure patient informs member of staff when urination has taken place	Ensures normal mechanism to urinate occurs and patient does not go into urinary retention
Draw back the curtains/open the door and dispose of equipment as per trust policy	Reduces environmental contamination Ensures accurate communication

(Cont'd)

Action	Rationale
Record urine output and when catheter removed	
Dispose of gloves and apron as pert trust policy Wash and dry hands thoroughly	Reduces the risk of infection

PROCEDURE: ADMINISTRATION OF ENEMAS

Action	Rationale
Explain and discuss the procedure with the patient Obtain consent	Ensures patient understanding and consent is valid and informed
Allow emptying of bladder; ensure bedpan/commode/toilet/toilet paper accessible; maintain privacy and dignity	Full bladder may cause discomfort Avoids unnecessary embarrassment In case there is a need to open bowels before the procedure has been completed
Warm the enema in a tray/jug of warm water	Heat is an effective stimulant of the plexi nerve in the intestinal mucosa and heating the enema to the body's temperature or above wont damage the intestinal mucosa
Draw the curtains/close the door, lie the patient on the left side with knees and buttocks flexed near the edge of the bed	Maintains privacy and dignity Position allows the ease of passage into the rectum by following the natural anatomy of the colon. Gravity aids the flow of the solution into the colon while flexing the knees ensures it is a more comfortable passage for the enema nozzle into the rectum
Place an incontinence pad under the patient's hip and buttocks	Avoids embarrassment if fluid is ejected prematurely Reduces the potential for infection
Wash and dry hands thoroughly Wear gloves and apron	Minimises risk of cross-infection
Place some lubricating jelly onto the nozzle of the enema	Lubricates the nozzle; prevents trauma to the anal and rectal mucosa by reducing the surface friction

Action	Rationale
Expel air and introduce the nozzle slowly 10–12.5 cms into the anal canal while separating the buttocks and informing the patient of what is happening	Introducing air into the colon bypasses the anal canal, causes distension of the wall, discomfort and increases peristalsis. Introducing the nozzle 10–12.5 cms bypasses the anal canal (which is 2.5–4.5 cms in length) and ensures the nozzle is in the rectum. Slow introduction minimises spasm of the intestinal wall
If a retention enema is administered, introduce the contents slowly and leave the bed elevated 45 degrees for as long as possible	Avoids increasing peristalsis while slow insertion of the contents means less pressure is exerted on the intestinal wall. Elevating the bed facilitates the retention of the enema
Retention enemas used for drug administration should be retained for a minimum of 30 minutes so ensure patient remains lying in the left lateral position with the foot of the bed elevated	Aids retention and absorption of the drug administered
If an evacuant enema is administered, introduce slowly by rolling from the bottom of the pack to introduce the contents Ask patient to retain for as long as possible	Rolling from the bottom of the pack prevents back flow; increases pressure on the rectal wall; distension and irritation of the bowel wall resulting in strong peristalsis and effective emptying of the bowel
Slowly withdraw the nozzle and clean the patient perianal area	Avoids reflex emptying of the rectum Promotes patient dignity and avoids excoriation
Ask patient to retain contents for 10–15 minutes before opening the bowels	For effective evacuation of the bowel
Ensure patient has access to call bell, bedpan/commode/toilet/toilet paper	Enhances patient comfort and dignity
Remove and dispose of equipment Wash and dry hands thoroughly as per trust policy	Minimises risk of cross-infection
Record enema given; its effects and results on charts/notes	Legal requirement; effective communication; monitors bowel function
Allow patient to wash their hands/sacral area if bowel open	Minimises risk of cross-infection

PROCEDURE: ADMINISTRATION OF SUPPOSITARIES

Action	Rationale
Explain and discuss the procedure with the patient and obtain consent If suppository medicated (e.g., paracetamol) ensure bowel is opened first	Ensures patient understanding and consent is informed and valid Ensures patient has full benefit of the medication/absorbed by the rectal mucosa and not expelled when bowels opened
Ensure privacy, dignity and bedpan/commode/toilet/toilet paper available	Avoids unnecessary embarrassment and in case of premature expulsion of the suppository, or rapid bowel evacuation
Lie patient on left side with knees flexed and buttocks near the edge of the bed	Ease of the passage into the rectum following natural anatomy of the colon Flexed knees reduces discomfort as suppository enters the anal canal
Place an incontinence pad under the patient hips and buttocks having drawn the curtains/closed the door	Avoids soiling of bed linen, potential infection and patient embarrassment if bowels open prematurely
Wash and dry hands thoroughly, wear gloves and apron	Reduces risk of cross-infection
Place lubricating jelly on blunt end of suppository; separate buttocks and insert blunt end 2–4 cms, while informing patient of its insertion	Lubrication reduces surface friction, eases insertion and avoids anal mucosal trauma Blunt end eases retention of the suppository
Clean patient perianal area once suppository inserted Ask patient to retain suppository for minimum 10–15 minutes	Promotes patient comfort, dignity and avoids excoriation Allows suppository to melt and release active ingredients
Leave patient in comfortable position with call bell Ensure access to bedpan/commode/toilet/toilet paper Ensure curtains drawn/door closed	Ensures patient privacy and dignity maintained
Remove, dispose of equipment; wash and dry hands thoroughly	Reduces risk of infection
Record administration of suppository, any effects and result	Legal requirement and effective communication Monitors bowel function

PROCEDURE: STOMA CARE

Action	Rationale
Explain and discuss the procedure with the patient and obtain consent	Ensures patient understands the procedure and gives their consent
Close the door/draw the curtains Ensure the patient is in a comfortable position and able to watch the procedure	Maintains privacy and dignity Allows for good access to the stoma for cleaning and securing the appliance
Use a small protective pad to protect the patient's clothing Wear gloves and apron	Avoids changing clothes or linen Prevents cross-infection
If a bag is the drainable type empty the contents first into a jug before removing the bag	Easy handling of the bag and prevents spillage
Remove spillage Peel adhesive off the skin with one hand while exerting gentle pressure on the skin with the other hand	Reduces trauma to the skin
Fold the appliance in two and place in a disposal bag	Ensures no spillage occurs and safe disposal according to environmental policy
Remove excess faeces or mucous from the stoma with a damp tissue	So the stoma and surrounding skin are clearly visible
Examine the skin and stoma for soreness, ulceration or other complications. If the stoma and skin are healthy and red in colour continue	Prevents complications or treatment of existing problems
If complications present inform senior nursing staff/medical team, document and treat as prescribed	Prevents further complications occurring
Wash the skin and stoma gently until clean	Promotes cleanliness and prevents skin excoriation
Dry the skin and stoma gently	Ensures the appliance will attach more securely
Measure the stoma using measuring guide, cut the appliance leaving 3 mm clearance and apply to the skin	Should provide skin with protection Aperture cut slightly larger that the stoma so the contents cannot cause skin damage and appliance doesn't rub the stoma

(Cont'd)

Action	Rationale
Dispose of the soiled tissue and used appliance in a disposable bag and place in an appropriate bin At home place the stoma bag in a bag, tie and dispose into the rubbish bin	Ensures safe disposal
Wash hands thoroughly after removing gloves and apron with bactericidal soap and water, or bactericidal alcohol hand rub	Prevents spread of infection by contaminated hands

References

Barton, R (2000) Intermittent Self Catheterisation, *Nursing Standard* 15(9): 1–9.

Black, PK (2000a) Practical Stoma Care, *Nursing Standard* 14(41): 47–55.

Black, PK (2000b) *Holistic Stoma Care*. Balliere Tindall, London.

Borwell, B (1997) Ileo-Anal Pouch Surgery and Its After Care, *Community Care* 3 (7): 15–20.

Bridgewater, SE (1999) Dietary Considerations. In P. Taylor (ed.) *Stoma Care in the Community. A Clinical Resource for Practitioners*. Nursing Times Books, London.

Brown, H and Randle, J (2005) Living With a Stoma: A Review of the Literature, *Journal of Clinical Nursing* 14 (1): 74–81.

Burch, J and Sica, J (2005) Stoma Care Accessories: An Overview of a Crowded Market, *British Journal Community Nursing* 10(4): 24–31.

Cadd, A et al. (2000) Assessment and Documentation of Bowel Care Management in Palliative Care: Incorporating Patient Preferences into the Care Regimen, *Journal of Clinical Nursing* 9: 228–235.

Chelvanayagam, S and Norton, C (2004) Nursing Assessment of Adults with Faecal Incontinence. In C Norton, and S Chelvanayagam (eds) *Bowel Continence Nursing*. Beaconsfield Publishers, Beaconsfield.

Davenport, K and Keeley, FX (2005) Evidence for the Use of Silver Alloy Coated Urethral Catheters, *Journal of Hospital Infection* 60(4): 298–303.

DH (1999) *Making a Difference – Strengthening the Nursing, Midwifery and Health Visiting Contribution to Health and Health Care*. DH, London.

DH (2000) *Good Practice in Continence Services*. HMSO, London.

DH (2001) *Essence of Care Document*. DH, London.

DH (2004) Bardex IC: Silver Alloy Coated Hydrogel Catheters. www.hpa.org.uk/infections/topicsaz/rapidreview/pdf/bardex2.pdf

Dougherty, L and Lister, S (2006) *The Royal Marsden Hospital Manual Clinical Nursing Procedures*, 6th edn. Blackwell Publishing, Oxford.

Doughterty, L and Lister, S (2008) *The Royal Marsden Hospital Manual Clinical Nursing Procedures*, *Student Edition*, 7th edn. Blackwell Publishing, Oxford.

Dunn, S et al. (2000) *Management of Short Term Indwelling Urethral Catheters to Prevent CAUTI in Hospitalised Patients. A Systematic Review*. The Joanna Briggs Institute of Evidence Based Nursing and Midwifery, Australia.

Fazio, VW and Wu, PS (1997) Surgical Therapy for Crohn's Disease of the Colon and Rectum, *Surgical Clinic North America* 77: 197–210.

Fillingham, S and Douglas, J (1997) *Urological Nursing*. Balliere Tindall, London.

Fillingham, S and Fell, S (2004) Urological Stomas. In S Fillingham and J Douglas (eds) *Urological Nursing*, 2nd edn. Balliere Tindall, London.

Heins, T and Ritchie, K (1985) *Beating Sneaking Poo*. ACT Health Authority, Canberra Publishing and Printing Co.

Hogan, CM (1998) The Nurses Role in Diarrhoea Management, *Oncology Nursing Forum* 25(5): 879–886.

King, D (2002) Determining the Cause of Diarrhoea, *Nursing Times* 98(23): 47–48.

Kirkwood, L (1999) Taking Charge, *Nursing Times* 95(6): 63–64.

Kyle, G et al. (2005) The Eton Scale: A Tool for Risk Assessment for Constipation, *Nursing Times* 101(18 Suppl): 50–51.

Kornblau, A et al. (2000) Management of Cancer Treatment Related Diarrhoea: Issues and Therapeutic Strategies, *Journal of Pain Symptom Management* 19(2): 111–119.

Moore, KN et al. (1993) Bacteruria in Intermittent Cathrterisation Users: The Effect of Sterile Verses Clean Reused Catheters, *Rehab Nurs* 18: 306–309.

Naish, W (2003) Intermittent Self Catheterisation for Managing Urinary Problems, *Professional Nurse* 18(10): 7–9.

NHS Modernisation Agency (2003) Essence of Care; Patient Focused Benchmarks for Clinical Governance. www.modern.nhs.uk/home/key/docs

NICE (2003) *Infection Control No 1 Standard Principles*. NICE, London.

NICE (2003a) *Infection Control: Prevention of Healthcare Associated Infections in Primary and Community Care*. NICE, London.

NMC (2007) *Guidance for the Introduction of the Essential Skills Clusters for Pre-Registration Nursing Programmes*. NMC, London.

Norton, C (1996) *Nursing for Continence,* 2nd edn. Beaconsfield Publishers, Beaconsfield.

Nugent, KP (1999) Intestinal Stomas. In CD Johnson and I Taylor (eds) *Recent Advances in Surgery* 22 Churchill Livingstone, Oxford.

Peate, I (2003) Nursing Role in the Management of Constipation: Use of Laxatives, *British Journal of Nursing* 12(19): 1130–1136.

Penfold, P (1999) Urinary Tract Infection in Patients with Urethral Catheters, *British Journal of Nursing* 8(6): 362–374.

Pomfret, IJ (2000) Catheter Care in the Community, *Nursing Standard* 22(14): 46–51.

Pratt, RJ et al. (2001) *Epic 1: The Development of National Evidence Based Guidelines for Preventing Hospital Acquired Infections In England Standard Principles: Technical Report*. Thames Valley University, London.

Price, B (1996) Practical Support Roles for Relatives of Stoma Patients, *Eurostoma* 16: 10–11.

RCN (2006) *Digital Rectal Exam and Manual Removal of Faeces: Guidance for Nurses*. RCN, London.

Robinson, J (2001) Urethral Catheter Selection, *Nursing Standard* 25(15): 39–42.

Royal College of Physicians (1995) Incontinence: Causes, Management and Provision of Services, *Journal of the Royal College of Physicians* London 29(4): 272–274.

Saint, S et al. (1999) Preventing Catheter Related Bacteriuria: Should We? Can We? How? *Archive of Internal Medicine* 159: 800–808.

Schaeffer, AJ (2002) Infections of the Urinary Tract. In PC Walsh et al. (eds) *Campbell's Urology*, 8th edn. Saunders, Philadelphia.

Sedar, J and Mulholland, SG (1999) Hospital Acquired Urinary Tract Infections Associated With the Indwelling Catheter, *Urology Clinics of North America* 26: 821–828.

Simpson, L (2001) Indwelling Urethral Catheters, *Nursing Standard* 15(46): 47–54.

Smith, S (2001) Evidence Based Management of Constipation on the Oncology Patient, *European Journal of Oncology Nursing* 5(1). 18 25.

Taylor, P (2000) Choosing the Right Stoma Appliance for a Colostomy, *Nurse Prescribing Community Nurse* 6(9): 35–38.

Taylor, P (2005) An Introduction to Stomas: Reasons for Their Formation, *Nursing Times* 101(29): 63–64.

Tenke, X et al. (2004) Prevention and Treatment of Catheter, Associated Infections: Myth or Reality? *EVA Update Series* 2: 106–115.

Thompson, MJ et al. (2003) Management of Constipation, *Nursing Standard* 18(14–16): 41–42.

Tortora, GJ and Grabowski, SR (2002) *Principles of Anatomy and Physiology*. John Wiley, New York.

Walker, S (2007) Elimination. In C Brooker and A Waugh (eds) *Foundations of Nursing Practice Fundmentals of Holistic Care*. Mosby, Edinburgh.

Walsh, M (1997) *Watson's Clinical Nursing and Related Sciences,* 5th edn. Balliere Tindall, Edinburgh.

Ward, V et al. (1997) Preventing Hospital Acquired Infections: Clinical Guidelines, *Public Health Laboratory Services*. PHLS, London.

Wilson, M (1998) Infection Control, *Professional Nurse Study Supplement* 13(5): S10 –S13.

Winn, C (1996) Catheterisation: Extending the Scope of Practice, *Nursing Standard* 10(52): 49–56.

Winn, C (1998) Complications with Urinary Catheters, *Professional Nurse Study Supplement* 10(52): S7–S10.

Winney, J (1998) Constipation, *Nursing Standard* 13(11): 49–56.

www. hed2.bupa.co.uk/fact_sheets/html/stoma_care

www.patient.co.uk

www.student.bmj.com/issues

www.surgical-tutor.org.uk/specialities/general/stoma

10

Administration of Medicines

Learning Outcomes

This chapter is designed to help you:

o   understand the guidelines and legislation pertaining to the administration of medicines
o   be aware of potential errors in the administration of medicines
o   be aware of issues concerning drug calculations
o   understand the principles of drug administration and acquire knowledge of the main routes used
o   understand the nurse's role and professional responsibilities.

Introduction

Drug administration is a major part of the nurse's role. The Audit Commission (2001) estimates that 40 per cent of nurses' time is spent dealing with medication. Doing so safely is of the utmost importance, as failure to administer medication to patients correctly can have dire consequences ranging from an allergic reaction to patient death. This chapter will examine the law and guidelines regarding administration of medicines, issues such as safe storage, the ordering and prescription of medicines, the essential skills required to administer medication, and how medication errors are handled.

Legislation and Guidelines

Drug administration is defined as the way medicines are selected, procured, delivered, prescribed, administered and reviewed, to optimise the contribution that medicines make to producing informed and desired outcomes of patient care (Audit Commission 2001). The professional role of the nurse involves the safe handling and administration of medicine. It also includes a need to ensure understanding by the patient (Luker and Wolfson 1999). NMC (2007: 26) clearly states that students need to 'ensure safe and effective practice through comprehensive knowledge of medicines, their actions, risks and benefits'.

The manufacture, safe storage, prescription and sales of medicines within the United Kingdom are subject to a number of regulations: they include the Medicines Act (1968), Misuse of Drugs Act (1971) and Misuse of Drugs Regulations (2001). There are also a number of professional regulations to be aware of, e.g., Guidelines for the Administration of Medicines (NMC 2004), The Code (NMC 2008), Guidelines for Records and Record Keeping (NMC 2005), Standards for Medicines Management (NMC 2008a) and Standards for Proficiency for Pre-Registration Nursing Education (NMC 2004a). The Medicinal Products: Prescription by Nurses Act (1992) has been enhanced by the publication of two further reports (DH 1998, DH 1999). Here the NMC (2007) Essential Skills Cluster document is of crucial importance for nursing students, who must be able to demonstrate competence in essential skills in order to progress from common foundation programme to branch and then onto the register. Increasingly, qualified nurses are able to prescribe drugs once they have undertaken specific training to do so.

Storing of Medication

MHRA (2001) provides recommendations regarding how to store medication at the appropriate temperature. Local trusts have used this document as a basis for producing their own policy. The Duthrie Report (DH 1988) states that medicines should be stored either in a locked cupboard, locked in a medicine trolley, in a locked section of a patient's bedside locker (patient's own drugs), or in a locked refrigerator (for any product to be stored at a temperature between two and eight degree celcius), while some are stored at room temperature away from direct sunlight (between 15–25 degrees celcius) or kept in the original packaging. Storing medicines at home involves consulting the manufacturer's instructions concerning storage, keeping refrigerated drugs away from raw food and keeping drugs away from children.

Controlled Drugs

Controlled drugs (CDs) are 'drugs of addiction which produce dependence' (Downie et al. 2003). The Misuse of Drugs Act (1971) and Misuse of Drugs Regulations (1985, amended in 2006 (DH 2006a)) regulate controlled drugs, so familiarity with these documents is required. The drugs are locked in an inner cupboard within a cupboard and the contents and CD register must be checked as per trust policy. A red light indicates when the cupboard is open while the register is kept as an accurate record of the contents of the CD cupboard. Keys for both cupboard and inner cupboard are held by the nurse in charge, separately from the main keys. Lost or stolen keys should be reported immediately to senior staff and local protocol followed.

Non-controlled drugs may ordered by a first level nurse or pharmacist using an order sheet. On receipt of the drugs, a first level nurse must check them against the order sheet for accuracy. For CDs a first level nurse completes a carbonised order form and the pharmacy dispenses the drug, which then has to be signed for before it leaves the pharmacy in a sealed package. On the ward, the CD must be checked by two level-one nurses against the order book. The volume to the stock should be recorded in the CD register. The pharmacist will keep a record of the CD ordered and the amount dispensed.

Table 10.1   *Reasons for medication errors*

Drug omission
Administering an unauthorised drug, i.e., not prescribed
Wrong dose being administered
Administered via the wrong route
Wrong time of administration
Poor maths skills in miscalculating the dose
Lack of knowledge regarding the drug administered
Tiredness due to increased workload
Interruption during the drug round, i.e., the nurse being called away
Unsupervised practice
Poor practice/procedure
Poor communication/documentation
Distraction.

(Brooker and Waugh 2007)

Medication Errors

NPSA (2007) defined a medication error as a 'preventable event that may cause or lead to inappropriate medication use or patient harm while the medication is in the control of the health professional, patient or consumer'. It is the most common and consistent type of error occurring in hospitals (Luk et al. 2008). The DH (2000) has highlighted how and why common drug errors occur. The Audit Commission (2001) found that medication errors account for one fifth of deaths due to all types of adverse reactions. Thomas et al. (2000) found that 35.1 per cent of adverse events involving medication were preventable. Lassetter and Warnick (2003) identified several types of medication errors. these included prescribing medication known to interact when administered together, prescribing a medication the patient was known to be allergic to, misreading or misinterpreting handwriting and abbreviations, confusing similar medications, not diluting a concentrated medication and omission error.

Medication errors arise for a number of reasons, as noted in Table 10.1. This is supported by a study undertaken by Cook et al. (2004). Following incidents in the NHS, NPSA (2007) published new recommendations in order to improve safety. If drug administration, following NMC and local policy guidelines, is well planned, the chance of errors can certainly be reduced. Critical care and paediatric areas are high risk areas for medication errors (Richardson 2008). This is because there are many different healthcare professionals at various stages of the administration of the medication process (e.g., ordering, prescribing, transcribing, verifying, dispensing, delivering and administering) (Raju et al. 1989, Viner et al. 1989).

If a medication error occurs, this may result in disciplinary action for the nurse concerned. There may be an investigation for professional misconduct, criminal charges or a civil case for **negligence**. Any medication error that does occur should be dealt with by reporting the incident: reporting errors can protect patients and staff and can also help to identify areas for improvement (Richardson 2008). Luk et al. (2008) suggest senior nursing staff manage medication errors with the nurse, patient and relatives concerned. When dealing with the nurse involved in the medication error, ethical principles of justice and the need for respect apply: the nurse must be treated fairly and not unjustly blamed for the error. The nurse should not be humiliated because an error has occurred (Luk et al. 2008). The reporting process involves informing senior staff, completing an incident report and undertaking an investigation – as opposed to simply apportioning blame or immediately instigating disciplinary processes.

Current policy states that clear records are required regarding the administration of medicines, as specified by government recommendations relating to safe medicine administration practice (DH 2000, NMC 2005). Only the most necessary drugs should be prescribed, i.e., those patients who have already been prescribed and require, for instance, insulin. Writing clearly on the prescription chart, prior to administering the medicine, in accordance with government recommendation and trust policy, is important to ensure the medication prescribed is administered safely. Any omission of medication must also be recorded with a reason provided, e.g., drug not available, patient refused.

NPSA (2007) advised that the risk of medication errors could be reduced by safer product designs (for example, of oral syringes). NPSA (2007) established seven priority areas to improve medication safety – increased reporting and learning from incidents, implementation of NPSA safe medication practice recommendations, improving staff skills for competencies, minimising dose errors, ensuring medicines are not omitted, ensuring the correct drug is given to the right patient and documenting any allergies.

Drug Calculations

Drug incidents cost an estimated £750 million per year to the NHS in England (NPSA 2007). On average, they result in an average of eight and a half additional days in hospital. Familiarity with trust policies and procedures, combined with a sound pharmacological knowledge base of drugs, is required on the part of nurses. This view is supported by Nicol and Thompson (2001), who viewed the administration of medicines as a key aspect of care requiring theoretical knowledge, numeracy, negotiation, patient teaching and reflective skills. A sound and comprehensive knowledge is required concerning the actions and effects of medicines, their interactions, why they are taken, how they are eliminated, doses, frequency and the action to take if doses are omitted. Such knowledge is known as **pharmacokinetics** (considers what effects the drug has on the body) and **pharmacodynamics** (how the body affects the drug with time, i.e., what the body does to the drug).

It is absolutely essential to be able to calculate drug dosages accurately and to be fully conversant with the units of drugs in current use (Watt 2003). The need is substantiated by Brown (2002), who found that nursing students were mathematically under-prepared regarding drug calculations. Brown (2002) stressed the importance of calculating dosages correctly and suggested that maths tests and remedial courses be held each semester during pre-registration courses.

LEARNING ACTIVITY 10.1

Select two patients from practice and find out:

- What medication(s) they have been prescribed?
- What the medication(s) are used for and their action(s)?
- What the normal dose would be for an adult and child?
- What the side effects and contraindications are?

Be sure to maintain patient confidentiality.

It is important to understand and have a working knowledge of formulae for complex calculations (Downie et al. 2003). To ensure the correct volume or quantity is administered, it may be necessary to have a second registered nurse to check the dose and minimise errors occurring (Richardson 2008), especially since many qualified nurses and students struggle with basic pharmacology and drug calculation. Incorrect drug calculations can cause medication errors and harm to the patient (or even death (DH 2000, O'Shea 1999)). DH (2004) aimed to improve nurses' drug calculation skills in order to reduce the number of drug errors in the NHS by 50 per cent by 2005, as it was discovered in practice that many nurses required support with ratios, percentages, fractions and they were sometimes unable to interpret information found in clinical areas into drug calculations (Hendry et al. 1999, Haigh 2002).

Most drugs are manufactured in a form that enables straightforward administration. Some are available in a variety of strengths. This helps to ensure that the prescribed dose can be safely and easily calculated and hence administered accurately. An international system of units (SI) is normally used in prescriptions (avoiding the use of decimal points), while International Units (IU) are used for some preparations, e.g., insulin, heparin.

Calculating the therapeutic safe dose of any medication is achieved by calculating weight and safe dose per kilogram or calculating the patient's body surface area. The dose is calculated using the metric system and described in units in this system. When calculating the dose required ensure the same units are used (e.g., grams or milligrams).

Box 10.2   Conversions and Formulae

1 kilogram (kg) = 1000 grams (g)
1 gram (g) = 1000 milligrams (mgs)
1 milligram (mgs) = 1000 micrograms (mcg)
1 litre (l) = 1000 millilitres (mls)
1 millilitre = 1000 microlitres

To convert large units to small units:

kilograms (kg) to grams (g) = × 1000
grams (g) to milligrams (mgs) = × 1000
milligrams (mg) to micrograms (mcg) = × 1000
micrograms (mcg) to nanograms (ng) = × 1000
litres (l) to millilitres (ml) = × 1000

To convert small units to large units:

grams (g) to kilograms (kg) = % 1000
milligrams (mg) to grams (g) = % 1000
micrograms (mcg) to milligrams (mg) = % 1000
nanograms (ng) to micrograms (mcg) = % 1000
millilitres (mls) to litres (l) = % 1000

(Cont'd)

To calculate the number of tablets or capsules required for administration the following formula is used:

$$\frac{\text{dose prescribed}}{\text{dose available}} = \text{number of tablets/capsules required}$$

For liquid preparations the following formula is used:

$$\frac{\text{dose prescribed} \times \text{volume available}}{\text{dose available}} = \text{volume to be administered (ml)}$$

To administer fluids a fluid administration set is required which administers the fluid as 'drops per min'. Crystalloid administration sets operate at 20 drops/ml; blood (large bore) sets operate at 15 drops/ml; burettes operate at 60 drops/ml. The following formula is used:

$$\frac{\text{flow rate}}{\text{(drops/min)}} = \frac{\text{volume of fluid (ml)} \times \text{set rate (no. of drops/ml)}}{\text{hours} \times 60 \text{ mins}}$$

For instance, 1 litre of saline is prescribed and to be infused over eight hours. Calculate the drip rate.

$$\frac{1000 \times 20}{8 \times 60} = \frac{20000}{480} = 41.6 \text{ OR } 42 \text{ drops/min}$$

Fluid infusions administered via volumetric pumps use the following formula:

$$\frac{\text{flow rate}}{\text{(ml/hour)}} = \frac{\text{volume of fluid}}{\text{time (hour)}}$$

For instance, 5000 mls of fluid is prescribed and to be infused over six hours. Calculate the drip rate:

$$\frac{500}{6} = 83.3 \text{ OR } 83 \text{ drops/hr}$$

For calculations based on body weight, prescription is expressed as mls per kg (ml/kg) or mg per kg (mg/kg). The following formula is used:

$$\frac{\text{weight (kg)} \times \text{dosage per day}}{\text{number of doses per day}} = \text{mg per dose}$$

For instance, a child weighing 16 kg is prescribed intravenous (IV) erythromycin for a severe infection. The dose is 50mg/kg/day in four doses:

$$\frac{16\text{kg} \times 50\text{mg/kg/day}}{\text{four doses/day}} = \frac{800}{4} = 200 \text{ mg/dose}$$

Therefore 200 mgs of erythromycin is administered four times a day.

To minimise the number of medication errors caused by miscalculating the dose, volume, or rate of administration, nurses and students need to be familiar with these formulae and the role they play in drug administration. DH (2004) provides guidance and recommendations of good practice for healthcare professionals, to enable them to examine their current practice and improve medication safety. This should be informed by an understanding of the NMC documents – NMC (2008) The Code, NMC (2005) Guidelines for Records and Record Keeping, NMC (2004) Administration of Medicines and NMC (2008a) Standards of Medicines Management. NMC (2008) states that nursing students must be competent in basic medicine calculations and administer medication safely under direct supervision.

LEARNING ACTIVITY 10.2

Mrs Gant is an 80 year old nursing home resident with Alzheimer's Disease. She has been diagnosed with right lower lobe pneumonia. When the nurse offers Mrs Gant her 14.00 antibiotics she shouts, 'I'm not taking that! Get out!'
   What is the most appropriate course of action?

LEARNING ACTIVITY 10.3

Joanne, aged 13, is currently in hospital receiving treatment for an infection. She is prescribed oral antibiotics three times a day. Staff Nurse Britton is doing the medication round and has dispensed Joanne's antibiotics.
   Joanne says she is going to the toilet, asks for the antibiotics to be left on the locker and says she will take them on her return.
   What should the nurse do?

Drug Administration

The aim of drug administration is to create therapeutic values while avoiding toxic levels of the drug. This requires monitoring treatment and side effects and recording any medication given or omitted. Medicines must always be administered in accordance with legislation, local trust policies and NMC guidelines.

Covert administration of any medication should be considered only in accordance with UKCC (2001) guidelines. These state that covert administration may only be carried out in some specific instances (e.g., if an individual who has actively refused the medication is judged not to have the capacity to understand the consequences of refusing). NMC (2008: 1) states that covert administration of medicines 'should not be confused with the administration against someone's will, which in itself may not be deceptive, but may be unlawful'.

Disguising medication constitutes deception, even if done with the best of intentions. NMC (2001a, 2001b, 2008a) states that 'by disguising medication in food and drink, the patient or client is being led to believe that they are not receiving medication when in fact they are' (p. 1). Disguising medication in food is acceptable under some circumstances, i.e., to prevent a patient who is incapable of informed consent from missing out on essential treatment (NMC 2001a, 2001b, 2008a).

Common law states that every person has the right to self determination and a duty of care by the practitioner. Every person is also presumed to have the mental capacity to consent to or refuse treatment unless the patient is unable to take in and retain the information regarding the medication, unable to understand the information, or unable to weigh up the information as part of the decision making process. Assessment is required of an individual's capacity to provide consent. Failure to obtain consent may result in a breach of human rights and the risk of assault. Consent may not, however, be possible from those with mental health problems, learning disabilities and children. Children under the age of 16 are generally considered to lack the capacity to consent to or refuse treatment or medication. Parents retain the right unless the child is considered to have an understanding and intelligence to make their own mind up. Consent may be obtained from a family member or guardian instead.

The Mental Heath Act (1983) makes provision for the compulsory detention and treatment in hospital of those with a mental health disorder (DH 2007). Continued assessment of the individual's ability to give consent or refuse medication is therefore essential. Detaining anyone under the Mental Health Act (1983) should only be considered as a last resort after all other options have been exhausted. For those who are detained under the Mental Health Act (1983), medication can be given against their wishes for the first three months of treatment or after, if sanctioned by a Second Opinion Appointed Doctor (SOAD).

The Mental Health Bill (DH 2006) replaced the 1983 Act Mental Health Act and was introduced in April 2008. The main areas of change included: making provision for people with serious and ongoing mental health problems to receive the necessary treatment, and to maintain their safety and that of the public; widening the range of healthcare professionals to perform roles identified in the 1983 Mental Health Act; reconfiguring legislation to reflect the multidisciplinary nature of modern mental health services and allowing them to act more rapidly and flexibly in response to service users' needs; and protecting the rights of people who do not have the capacity to provide consent and whose circumstances are not covered by the 1983 Mental Health Act.

Routes of Administration

Medicines may be administered via various routes. These may be divided into two main categories – systemic and local. Common systemic routes are oral, **sublingual/buccal**, inhalation, and injection, while common local routes are inhalation and topical. First, check information on the prescription chart, select the medication and check the expiry date, empty the prescribed dose into the lid of the bottle and then into the medicine pot. Liquid medicine should be measured using a specialist oral syringe, administered immediately and documented on the prescription chart according to the trust policy.

Always check that you have the right patient (check their name band), right drug, right dose, administered via the right route at the right time and that the drug has had the right preparation. Also ensure that the right documentation is completed. Provide explanations of the drug being administered to allay patient anxieties, having first ascertained any allergies and gained consent.

REFER TO PROCEDURE: ORAL DRUG ADMINISTRATION

For children, always keep medicines out of reach and ensure drug dosages are prescribed according to age, body weight, body surface area or a combination of all of these. To prevent drug errors, all calculations must be checked, especially when using calculators. The NMC (2004) states 'the use of calculators to determine the volume or quantity of medication should not act as a substitute for arithmetical knowledge and skill'. If the prescribed dose is less than one millilitre (1 ml), an oral syringe should be used as it allows for a more accurate dose to be administered and the medicine should not be diluted into bottle feeds or other liquids.

Sugar-free liquid preparations are preferred for children, while injections should be avoided whenever possible. Infants, children and young people are constantly changing physically, metabolically and psychologically (Watt 2003). They metabolise, excrete and react to drugs differently to adults (Kanneh 2002) as plasma proteins in children are lower compared to that of adults. Changes in pharmacokinetics also occur at various times of child development (e.g., puberty), so nurses need a comprehensive understanding of the actions and effects of all medication taken by children when administering medication.

Psychological preparation of the child and family for the administration of medicines, knowledge and information of any previous drug reactions, and a joint decision making process, all make for successful administration of medication. This is especially important for the young, children or adults with a learning disability, in order to gain their cooperation.

Oral administration of prescribed medication includes tablets, capsules and liquids. Once swallowed the drug is usually absorbed from the lower intestine. Patients who experience difficulty in swallowing tablets may benefit from liquid formulations. Some tablets can be enteric coated or slow release. Avoid crushing them: this increases adverse drug reaction and toxicity (Miller and Miller 2000). Liquid formulation is certainly the preferred route for children and infants wherever possible, but can leave an unpleasant taste in the mouth (for instance, in the case of phenobarbitone syrup), so it is helpful to provide a drink or food after administration.

When administering liquid medication in infants use the following procedure to prevent aspiration: hold the child in the semi-reclining position, place the medication in the mouth with a spoon, dropper, syringe (following the manufacturer's instructions) or cup beside their tongue, and release the liquid slowly. Using a cup or spoon is useful to retrieve medicine from the chin lost due to natural outward tongue thrust (Watt 2003). Water, protective clothing and tissues can also prevent the child choking or aspirating.

For medicines not intended for swallowing, sublingual (under the tongue)/buccal (i.e., between the upper lip and gum, cheek) administration allows for rapid absorption of medicines into the blood vessels and mucous membrane in the mouth (for instance, glycerol trinitrate (GTN) spray). If the patient has a dry mouth, moisten the mouth before placing the tablet in the mouth.

Rapid absorption can also be achieved via rectal administration for some therapeutic drug administration (e.g., per rectum (PR) paracetamol) and for evacuation of the rectum (e.g., suppository or enema). The absorptive surface area of the rectum is small but the blood supply allows for a rapid absorption (Downie et al. 2006). (This is further explained in Chapter 8.)

This route may be used when patients complain of nausea and vomiting and are unable to swallow, when irritation of the upper gastrointestinal tract occurs, or when administering drugs to a local site (e.g., corticosteroids for irritable bowel syndrome). Pessaries may be administered into the vagina (e.g., nystatin pessaries for thrush (candida albicans)).

Inhaled medication is introduced directly for local action (e.g., bronchodilators to relieve bronchospasm) in respiratory conditions. The action is rapid and high concentrations can be delivered via inhaler devices designed to deliver drug particles to the small airways. Devices used include metered dose inhalers (ventolin), holding chambers or spacers (dry powder inhalers). Nebulisers are administered for acute respiratory problems and deliver a solution of the drug as a fine mist for patients to inhale through a mask or mouthpiece. The choice of device used will affect the chance of success as an uncooperative or distressed child may prevent successful treatment. Spacers, dry powder inhalers and metered dose inhalers are among the devices that may be used.

Topical medications are those applied to the surface area of the body. They include administration of creams, ointments, local anaesthetics and lotions for dermatological conditions. Instillations and irrigations (applied into body cavities or orifices), transdermal patches and liquid medicines prescribed are used to deliver medicines to produce systemic effects for a prolonged period (e.g., hormones, opioids, nicotine patches).

For an ear condition (e.g., to soften ear wax prior to irrigation or syringing) relieving inflammation or infections, lie the patient down or sit them up with the head tilted back and toward their opposite shoulder. Pull the projecting pinna (ear) upwards and back for adults; down and back for children and release upon administering ear drops. Ensure the patient keeps their head in position for between one and two minutes which allows the medication to enter the external auditory canal and the eardrum. The patient can then sit back upright again. Any excess fluid may need to be cleared away.

Administering optic, otic and nasal medication is not normally painful for the patient, though it can cause an unpleasant sensation. For children, lie the patient down and ask them to look up or tilt their head back. For small children, holding them close to the parent/carer's body may be required to minimise their limbs flailing. Therefore trust, cooperation, explanation and direction are required from and for the child and family for successful administration. Restraining techniques may be employed to immobilise the child's head (Watt 2003a).

After administration, ensure that the patient is comfortable, remove and dispose of the equipment used, document the administration of the medicine, ensure the patient knows why the medication was given, note when the medication takes effect and monitor for any side effects. If the patient has any swallowing difficulties, document and report them and consider alternative routes of administration. For example, if difficulties are faced in swallowing tablets, consider the prescription and administering of liquid medication instead, since it may prove easier to swallow.

Professional Responsibilities

Nurses are responsible for the correct administration of prescribed medication to patients in their care, in accordance with NMC (2008). It is the responsibility of the nurse when administering medicines to consider the patient's age (i.e., does the individual understand why the medication is required), past medical history (for example, is the individual on any other medication), whether the patient has a history of reacting to medication, the diagnosis (for example, if the individual is diabetic) and whether the patient consented to treatment. Also, the nurse should consider whether the patient has taken the medication prescribed before and how the patient takes the medication normally (e.g., orally). Other considerations include whether the patient has any allergies (e.g., to penicillin), whether there are any potential side effects (e.g., anaphylaxis), who administers the medicine, whether there are any contraindications to taking the medication, whether the appropriate medicine is being administered in the appropriate dose and in the appropriate formulation (e.g., liquid form) and whether it is administered by the appropriate route (i.e., oral, PR, IV). Patients should be monitored for side effects and response to treatment. Any adverse reactions should be reported (Sexton 1999).

When administering medication to children an understanding and a knowledge of child development and growth is required, as this will impact upon the dose prescribed, administered and drug interaction. Oral medication is usually administered in a sweetened form to make the medication more palatable. Covert administration of any medication in food, milk or juice can result in developing an unpleasant association with the food in question, with the result that the child refuses to eat or drink it in the future. Therefore, psychological approaches need to be considered when administering medication.

When administering an injection, one might encounter fear, needle phobia and anticipated pain on the part of the patient. In these circumstances, consider using an alternative, e.g., oral medication. If an injection is the only option (as for insulin administration), emla cream and demonstration on a toy prior to administration may be required. After demonstrating an injection, praise and cuddle the toy and speak softly to help dispel the association of pain and injections. This should be repeated when administering an injection to a child.

Summary

Nursing practice is underpinned by legislation that nurses must be aware of and adhere to. They must also be aware and familiarise themselves with the actions and side effects of drugs commonly used, and their professional responsibilities regarding drug administration according to law, national regulations and local trust policy.

PROCEDURE: ORAL DRUG ADMINISTRATION

Action	Rationale
Wash your hands	To minimise risk of cross-infection
Check the drug chart to ensure the medication is due and not already given	Meets legal requirements, hospital policy and NMC guidelines

(Cont'd)

Action	Rationale
Before administering the drug check the prescription chart for i the drug ii the dose iii date and time of administration iv dilutent as appropriate v validity of the prescription vi signature of the doctor vii is the prescription legible?	Ensures patient is given the correct drug Protects the patient from harm Complies with NMC (2005) Guidelines for Administration
Select the required medication, check the expiry date and empty dose into the container	Expiry date indicates drug no longer effective as drugs deteriorate with storage Minimises risk of cross-infection
Take the medication and prescription chart to the patient, check their identity, allergies and administer the medication with a glass of water	Ensures the medication is administered to the correct patient
Administer irritant drugs with meals/snacks, e.g., as with non-steroidal anti-inflammatory drugs (NSAIDs)	Breaking may cause incorrect dosage being given, gastrointestinal irritation or destruction of the drug
Don't break the tablet unless scored and it is appropriate to do so	Absorption rate is altered if chewed
Swallow slow release/enteric coated tablets; *do not* chew	Allows correct absorption of the drug
Sublingual drugs are administered under the tongue Buccal drugs are administered between the gums and cheek	More accurate than 5 ml spoon Ensures the correct dose is administered
Administering liquids to babies/young children, oral syringe should be used Place small amounts into the infants mouth For liquid controlled drugs, e.g., oramorph an oral syringe should be used	Prevents injury to the mouth and eliminates danger of choking Ensures the dose is administered and prevents the child spitting it out
Place the tip of the syringe towards the side of the mouth slowly inserting the contents towards the inside of the cheek If the child is uncooperative, place the end of the barrel between the teeth, or offer the choice of using a spoon	Prevents injury to the mouth and eliminates danger of choking Ensures dose is administered and prevents the child spitting it out/aspirating

Action	Rationale
Dilute oral medication if indicated with a small amount of water	Readily available if diluted in water. If a large amount of water is used the child may refuse to drink the entire amount and receive only a fraction of the prescribed medication
Record the administration on the prescription chart	Ensures effective communication that medication has been given

References

Audit Commission (2001) *A Spoonful of Sugar: Medicines Management in the NHS Hospital*. Audit Commission, London.

Brooker, C and Waugh, A (2007) *Foundations of Nursing Practice. Fundamentals of Holistic Care*. Mosby, Edinburgh.

Brown, DL (2002) Does 1 + 1 Equal 2? A Study of the Mathematic Competencies of Associate Degree Nursing Students, *Nurse Educator* 27(3): 132–135.

Cook, AF et al. (2004) An Error by Any Other Name, *American Journal of Nursing* 104: 32–43.

DH (1988) *The Duthrie Report*. DH, London.

DH (1998) *Review of Prescribing, Supply and Administration of Medicines. A Report on the Supply and Administration of Medicines Under Group Protocols*. Crown Two HMSO, London.

DH (1999) *Review of Prescribing, Supply and Administration of Medicines. Final Report*. Crown Three HMSO, London.

DH (2000) *An Organisation with a Memory*. DH, London.

DH (2004) *Building a Safer NHS for Patients: Improving Medication Safety*. The Stationary Office, London.

DH (2006) *Mental Health Bill*. DH, London.

DH (2006a) *Misuse of Drugs Regulations*. DH, London.

DH (2007) The *Mental Health Act 1983*. www.dh.gov.uk

Downie, G et al. (2003) *Calculating Drug Doses Safely*. Elsevier, London.

Haigh, S (2002) How to Calculate Drug Dosage Accurately: Advice for Nurses, *Professional Nurse* 18(1): 54–57.

Hendry, G et al. (1999) Construction and Problem Based Learning, *Journal of Further and Higher Education* 23(3): 359–371.

Kanneh, A (2002) Paediatric Pharmacological Principles: An Update Part 3: Pharmacokinetics: Metabolism and Excretion, *Paediatric Nursing* 14(10): 36–43.

Lassetter, JH and Warnick, ML (2003) Medical Errors, Drug-Related Problems and Medication Errors, *Journal Nurs Care Quartley* 18: 175–181.

Luker, K and Wolfson, D (1999) Introduction. In K Luker and D Wolfson (eds) *Medicines Management for Clinical Nurses*. Blackwell Science, Oxford.

Luk, LA et al. (2008) Nursing Management of Medication Errors, *Nursing Ethics* 15(1): 28–38.

Medicines Act (1968) HMSO, London.

Medicinal Products: Prescription by Nurses Act (1992)

Mental Health Act (1983) HMSO, London.

MHRA (2001) *Recommendations on the Control and Monitoring of Storage and Transportation Temperatures of Medicinal Products.* www.mhra.gov.uk

Miller, D and Miller H (2000) To Crush or Not to Crush, *Nursing* 30(2): 51–52.

Misuse of Drugs Act (1971) HMSO, London.

Misuse of Drugs Regulations (2001) HMSO, London.

Nicol, M and Thompson, B (2001) Cause of Medication Errors Part II, *Nursing Progress* 8: 9–11.

NMC (2001a) *Covert Administration of Medicines Can be Justified.* Press Statement 5th Sept, NMC, London.

NMC (2001b) *UKKC Position Statement on the Covert Administration of Medicines – Disguising Medicine In Food and Drink.* NMC, London.

NMC (2004b) *Code of Professional Conduct: Standards of Conduct, Performance and Ethics.* NMC, London.

NMC (2004) *Guidelines for Administration of Medicines.* NMC, London.

NMC (2004a) *Preparation for Pre-Registration Nurse Education.* NMC, London.

NMC (2005) *Guidelines for Records and Record Keeping.* NMC, London.

NMC (2007) *Guidance for the Introduction of the Essential Skills Clusters for Pre-Registration Nursing Programmes.* NMC, London.

NMC (2008) *The Code: Standards.* NMC, London.

NMC (2008a) *Standards of Medicines Management.* NMC, London.

NPSA (2007*) Safety in Doses: Improving the Use of Medications in the NHS.* www.npsa.nhs.uk

NPSA (2007) *Healthcare Risk Assessment Made Easy.* NPSA, London.

Raju, TNK et al. (1989) Medication Errors in Neo-Natal and PICU, *Lancet* 2: 374–376.

Richardson, R (ed.) (2008) *Clinical Skills for Student Nurses Theory, Practice and Reflection.* Reflect Press, Devon.

O'Shea, E (1999) Factors Contributing to Medication Errors: A Literature Review, *Journal of Clinical Nursing* 8: 496–504.

Sexton, J (1999) The Nurses' Role in Medicines Administration – Legal and Procedural Framework. In K Luker and D Wolfson (eds) *Medicines Management for Clinical Nurses.* Blackwell Science, Oxford.

Thomas, EJ et al. (2000) Incidence and Types of Adverse Events and Negligent Care in Utah and Colorado, *Medical Care* 38: 261–271.

UKCC (2001) *Position Statement on the Covert Administration of Medicines: Disguising Medicine in Food and Drink.* UKCC, London.

Viner, MJ et al. (1989) Drug Errors and Incidents in a Neo-Natal ICU, *American Journal Dis Child* 143: 737–740.

Watt, S (2003) Safe Administration of Medicines to Children: Part 1, *Paediatric Nursing* 15(4): 40–43.

Watt, S (2003a) Safe Administration of Medicines to Children: Part 2, *Paediatric Nursing* 15(5): 40–44.

11

Administration of Injections

Learning Outcomes

This chapter is designed to help you:

○ be aware of risks and safety considerations associated with the administration of injections
○ understand the legal and ethical considerations associated with the administration of injections
○ learn about common equipment used for subcutaneous and intramuscular injections.

Introduction

An injection can be described as the act of giving medication by use of a syringe and needle (Dougherty and Lister 2006). Injections are considered the appropriate route for drug administration when fast onset of action is required, patients who are nil by mouth, where the digestive enzymes would render the drug inactive (e.g., with insulin), long term release of the drug is necessary, e.g., depot injections (Brooker and Waugh 2007), or other routes may be contraindicated or impaired, e.g., patients maybe nil by mouth.

Administering injections have several disadvantages. These include arousing fear, anxiety and pain on the part of the patient. There are also safety issues associated with injections, including the risk of bruising, haematoma, sciatic nerve damage, drug reaction, accidental administration to the wrong tissue, abscess, tissue necrosis, cellulites, granuloma and lipohypertrophy. The disadvantages may be minimised by adopting effective interpersonal skills and good technique when administering the injection.

When administering an injection the equipment used includes syringes (which may be standard or 'luer lock') and are available in a variety of sizes (1–50 ml), while blunt and filter needles are available for 'drawing up', with needles varying in gauge (21–25G) and length. Needle gauge refers to the diameter of the needle's lumen and the size depends on the type of injection to be administered (orange 25G needles are used for S/C injections; green 21G or blue 23G for I/M injections depending upon muscle mass).

To gain experience in the administration of injections the NMC (2007) states students must be able to 'administer medication safely under direct supervision by injection' and it is the nurse's responsibility for the correct administration of the medication, for recording its administration and for supervising the student nurse. Any error must be recorded and reported according to trust policy (NMC 2004, NMC 2005). It is essential to follow guidelines, manufacturers' instructions and trust policies when administering injections.

LEARNING ACTIVITY 11.1

A nurse smells alcohol on a colleague's breath. Later in the evening the colleague asks for assistance when giving an injection. The nurse observes that her colleague's hand is shaking, is unable to landmark safely and the colleague doesn't appear to be able to focus on the task. What is the best intervention?

Subcutaneous (S/C) injections are administered into the fat and connective tissue that underly the dermis. They provide slower or sustained absorption into the subcutaneous fat or connective tissue lying between the muscles and skin. They are made using an orange (25G) needle, which allows a maximum of two millilitres (2 mls) to be administered, at an angle of insertion of 90 degrees (though for thin emaciated patients, an angle of 45 degrees may be necessary). With the introduction of shorter needles, King (2003) recommends insulin injections be given at an angle of 90 degrees.

The 'skin pinch' approach is adopted to lift the S/C tissue away from the underlying tissue. This helps ensure the medication is not inadvertently given intramuscularly. There is no need to aspirate as piercing a blood vessel is very rare (Peragallo-Dittko 1997), while aspirating heparin increases the risk of haematoma formation and pain. Sites used to administer S/C injections are lateral aspects of the upper arm, lateral aspects of the upper thigh and umbilical region of the abdomen.

REFER TO PROCEDURE: ADMINISTRATION OF SUBCUTANEOUS INJECTIONS

Intramuscular (I/M) injections are injected deep into the well perfused muscle, resulting in rapid systemic absorption. Use a green (21G) or blue (23G) needle, inserted at a 90 degree angle, allowing a maximum of five millilitres (5 mls) to be administered for adults and larger children and between one and two millilitres (1–2 mls) for infants (because their muscle mass is less than those of adults) (Workman 1999). The 'muscle bunch' technique allows the nurse to feel for muscle mass and decide the appropriate needle size to be used, while the 'Z track' approach creates a 'seal' over the track of injected medication, thereby causing less pain, preventing seepage and reducing incidence of the pain.

REFER TO PROCEDURE: ADMINISTRATION OF INTRAMUSCULAR INJECTIONS

Intramuscular injections allow various sites to be used. They include the deltoid muscle (for vaccinations and older children), dorsogluteal or upper outer quandrant of the buttock, due to the large amount of **adipose tissue** located here. Medication often remains here in the adipose tissue rather than the muscle so an appropriate length of needle is required, depending upon the size of the adult (Workman 1999, Greenway and Hainsworth 2004). Royal College of Paediatrics and Child Health (2002) do not advocate this site for children except when a large volume of fluid is to be injected. Other sites used include ventrogluteal (which avoids sciatic nerve damage), vastus lateralis muscle (used for children and infants after seven months of age), rectus femoris (rarely used for adults, but easily accessible for self administration or for infants) or quadriceps muscles (used for infants and young children).

Controversy surrounds the need to clean the skin prior to administering an injection. The use of alcohol swabs and cleaning the skin will depend on the local trust policy. If the trust policy advocates cleaning the skin, use an alcohol wipe, clean for 30 seconds and always leave 30 seconds for the skin to dry to allow adequate skin disinfection (Workman 1999). Downie et al. (2000) recommend immunosuppressed patients should have their skin cleaned as they may become infected by a relatively small number of pathogens. Always wash hands and use the non-touch technique when administrating injections, whether or not alcohol wipes are used.

Never re-sheath needles. To prevent needle stick injuries, dispose immediately of the needle and syringe into sharps containers. Ensure that you know the trust's policy regarding needle stick injury procedure. Children may associate an injection with a punishment (this may also explain why some adults also fear injections). Children receiving anticoagulants or with thrombocytopenia should not receive intramuscular injections. When administering injections to children under five years of age, they should be held firmly. Those between five and 12 require support, but should not be overpowered, while those over 12 should have their feelings recognised.

LEARNING ACTIVITY 11.2

Katie Morgan is a lively three year old who has just started at playschool for two mornings per week. She seems fearless and climbs to the top of all the play equipment. Katie doesn't talk very much and is slow to react to instructions from the play leaders. She seems to prefer to play on her own. One day, while climbing on the play equipment, Katie falls and is admitted to hospital. On admission Katie is in severe pain as indicated by the facial expressions (grimaces). Katie's mother arrives and is very upset and anxious that Katie has hurt herself and that she is in severe pain and requires analgesia for the pain. The analgesia is to be administered by an injection, which Katie is afraid of.

1 What information do (i) Katie and (ii) her mother require?
2 Are there alternative ways the analgesia can be administered?

LEARNING ACTIVITY 11.3

Gavin Davis, a 21 year old, has been living in a house for the past three years with four other male residents, all of whom have Down's Syndrome (Gavin included). The residents all help to undertake the chores under the supervision of the trained nurses.

Gavin works part time collecting trolleys from the car park of the local supermarket three mornings a week. One day Gavin accidentally cuts his hand at work. This requires sutures and a tetanus injection. Gavin is advised not to return to work until his hand has healed.

Given Gavin's learning disability (i.e., Down's Syndrome) how would you ensure (i) that he understands what is occurring and (ii) that he has his injection?

When administering injections, it is important to consider safety factors in order to minimise the risk of physical complications. It is necessary to know the drug, know what it is being taken for, and what its potential side effects are. It is also necessary to know the patient, the medication they are taking, and what allergies they may have, and to know the local trust's anaphylaxis policy. It is important to adopt standard precautions (e.g., hand washing) and use a non-touch technique.

Choosing an injection site is dependent upon the patient's age; health and muscle mass (as there is less muscle mass in the older and emaciated person); anatomical landmarks; absorption rate; volume to be administered; patient choice; and manufacturer's recommendation. This is because of the initial reasons identified for administrating medication via an injection, and to prevent discomfort and harm to the patient due to poor injection technique. Areas characterised by bruising, inflammation, infection, swelling, oedema, redness, scars, wounds, skin lesions or liphypertrophy should be avoided, as some drugs are likely to cause irritation and poor absorption. The drug may therefore need to be diluted in a greater volume of diluent. Microbes on the hand contribute to hospital-acquired infections (Weinstein 2007) so administration of an injection requires strict aseptic technique, hand washing and drying.

Summary

Complete, accurate documentation is essential as it is not only a legal requirement, but also serves to record the medication is given and the site where the injection was administered (thus helping to ensure rotation of the injection sites). Nurses must be aware of the legislation underpinning practice, safe administration of injections and disposal of equipment in accordance with local trust policy, and the action and side effects of drugs commonly administered.

Activity 1　Injection Technique

Label the following diagrams.

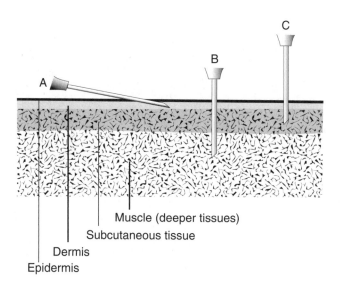

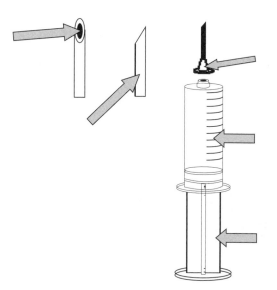

Activity 2

Subcutaneous injection sites

Circle the sites
that can be
used for SC
injection
administration

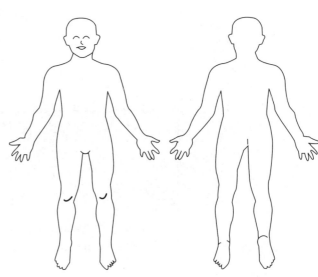

Intramuscular injection sites

Circle the sites
that can be
used for IM
injection
administration

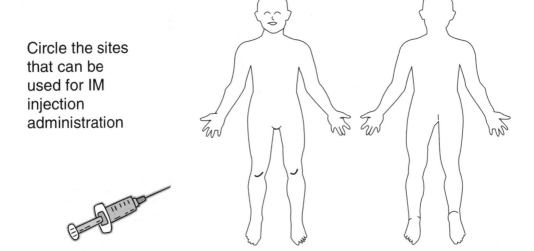

Activity 3

Complete the following table.

Type of Injection	Needle Size (gauge)	Colour
Drawing Up		
Subcutaneous		
Intramuscular		

Activity 4

Consider the interpersonal skills you might use when caring for a patient with a needle phobia.

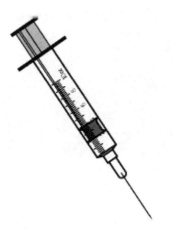

Activity 5

Review the following diagrams.
These show how to locate muscles used for IM injection administration.
With your partner discuss what the advantages and disadvantages of each might be.

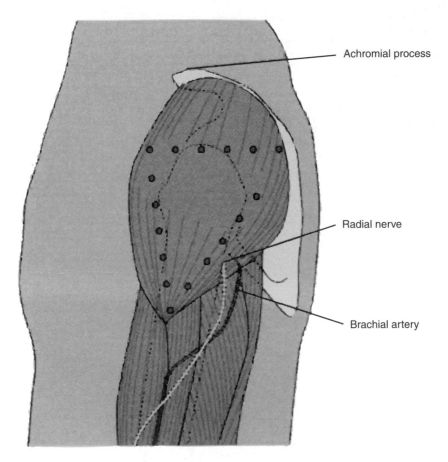

Achromial process

Radial nerve

Brachial artery

Deltoid

Picture taken from: Workman, B. 1999 Safe Injection Techniques, *Nursing Standard* 13(39): 47–53.

- Upper arm therefore easy access
- Densest part can be found by identifying the acromial process and the point on the lateral arm in line with the axilla
- Site the needle approx 2.5 cms below the acromial process
- Avoid radial nerve and brachial artery
- Ask patient to put hand on hip to relax the muscle
- Give up to 1 ml max.

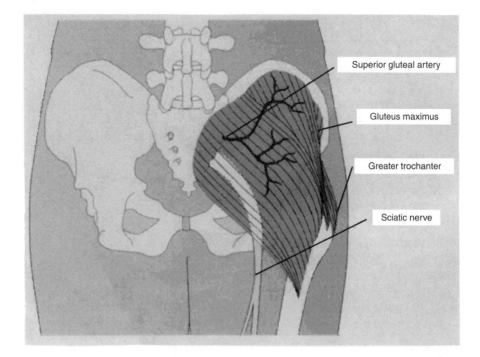

Superior gluteal artery

Gluteus maximus

Greater trochanter

Sciatic nerve

Dorsogluteal: carries risk of sciatic nerve damage

Picture taken from: Greenway, K. (2004) Using the Ventrogluteal Site for Intramuscular Injection, *Nursing Standard* 3(18): 39–42.

- Draw an imaginary horizontal line across from the top of the cleft in the buttocks to the greater trochanter of the femur
- Then draw an imaginary vertical line midway along the first line ...
- The location is the upper outer quadrant of the upper outer quadrant
- Avoids the sciatic nerve and the superior gluteal artery
- Can give up to 4 ml
- Ask patient to slightly flex legs to relax the muscle
- Has the lowest absorption rate.

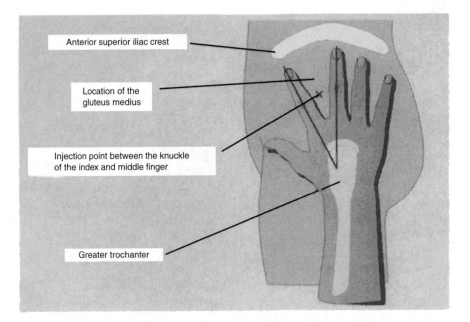

Anterior superior iliac crest

Location of the gluteus medius

Injection point between the knuckle of the index and middle finger

Greater trochanter

Ventrogluteal

Picture taken from: Greenway, K. 2004 Using the Ventrogluteal Site for Intramuscular Injection, *Nursing Standard* 3(18): 39–42.

- Uses the gluteus medius muscle
- No reported complications
- Avoids all major nerves and blood vessels
- Place the palm of your hand on the greater trochanter of the patient's hip (left hand to right hip, right hand to left hip)
- Extend your index finger to touch the anterior superior iliac crest
- Stretch your middle finger to form a V as far as possible along the iliac crest
- Instert the needle in the middle of the V
- Up to 4 ml volume can be given.

Recommended site for all IM injections

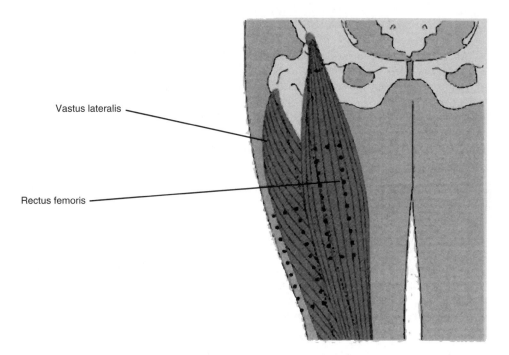

Vastus Lateralis

Picture taken from: Workman, B. 1999 Safe Injection Techniques, *Nursing Standard* 13(39): 47–53.

- Uses quadriceps muscle on the outer side of the femur
- Traditionally used for children but it is argued that the ventrogluteal site is better after seven months of age
- Over use of this muscle can result in muscle atrophy and femoral nerve damage
- Locate by measuring a hand's breadth laterally down from the greater trochanter and a hands breadth up from the knee
- Indentify the middle third of the muscle as the injection site
- Up to 5 ml volume can be given.

Rectus Femoris

- Uses anterior quadriceps muscle
- Easily accessed for self administration
- Located at the middle third of the anterior thigh
- Up to 5 ml can be given.

Drug Administration Workshop

- What is the name of the NMC booklet that gives advice to nurses about drug administration?
- When was it last updated?
- List five things that you should check/be sure of before administering a medicine to a patient/client?
- Name and date two pieces of legislation that relate to drug administration, safety and storage?
- How should the following be secured/stored in a clinical area?

  - controlled drug (CD)
  - medicines other than CD
  - emergency drugs
  - lotions.

- Where do you record information regarding storage and administration of controlled drugs (CD)?
- Name the sites on the body where the following injections can be given and at what angle should each type of injection be given – intramuscular, subcutaneous?
- Name four other routes by which medication can be given?
- For the following medication – paracetamol, tramadol, amoxicillin, find out

  - what the drug is used for and its action
  - what is the normal daily dose for an adult and child
  - what are the side effects and contraindications.

- What is amoxicillin used for and list three side effects.
- List four opioids and give two side effects.
- Name a specific reversing agent for diamorphine.

Drug Calculations

1) A child is prescribed 12 mg of gentamycin by injection. What volume is required for this dose if the stock ampoule contains 20 mg/2 mls?
2) A patient is prescribed morphine 7.5 mgs. What is the volume required if the stock ampoule contains 10 mg/2 mls?
3) 500 mls of normal saline is to be infused over a period of three hours. Calculate the required infusion rate for delivery of this prescription.
4) A patient requires 1 gram of amoxicillin which is available in 250 mg tablets. How many tablets are required for a single dose?
5) Calculate the volume of erythromycin required for a single dose if a patient weighing 60 kgs is prescribed 40 mg/kg/day in four doses.
6) 450 mls of blood is to be infused over three hours. At what number of drops per min should the transfusion be set?
7) What volume of salbutamol nebuliser solution is required if a patient is to receive 2.5 mgs? The stock solution contains 5 mg/2.5 mls.
8) A child is to receive 250 mgs of amoxicillin. The stock syrup contains 125 mgs in 5 mls. Calculate the volume of syrup to be given.

9) An elderly gentleman requires 1 g of paracetamol liquid as he cannot swallow. It is available in a suspension of 250 mg/5 mls. How many mls does he require?

10) A child weighing 15 kg requires trimethoprim. The total daily dose is 4 mg/kg to be given in two equal doses. Calculate a single dose.

PROCEDURE: ADMINISTRATION OF SUBCUTANEOUS INJECTIONS

Action	Rationale
Explain and discuss the procedure with the patient and obtain consent	Ensures patient understanding and that consent is informed and valid
Check the drug chart to ensure the medication is due and not already given	Meets legal requirements, hospital policy and NMC guidelines
Consult prescription chart and ascertain: the drug the dose date and time of administration dilutent as appropriate time of administration validity of the prescription signature of the doctor is the prescription legible?	Ensures patient is given the correct drug Protects the patient from harm Complies with NMC (2005) Guidelines for Administration
Close the door/draw the curtains and remove appropriate clothing Choose the site for injection and place the patient in the required position	Allows access to the chosen site and gains access for injection Maintains privacy, dignity and comfort
Choose the correct needle size	Minimises the risk of missing subcutaneous tissue and minimises pain
Pinch the skin into a fold	Elevates subcutaneous tissue and lifts adipose tissue away from underlying muscle
Insert the needle into the skin at 45–90 degree angle and release the pinched skin No need to withdraw the plunger and inject slowly	Injecting the medication into compressed tissue irritates the nerve fibres and causes discomfort It is unlikely the blood vessels are punctured
Withdraw the needle rapidly and apply pressure at the bleeding point	Prevents haematoma formation and backtracking
Ensure patient is comfortable and report abnormalities	Promotes comfort
Record administration on prescription chart	Maintains accurate record keeping
Dispose of sharp and non-sharp waste in accordance with trust policy, e.g., sharps into sharps container	Ensures safe disposal, avoids laceration and other injury

PROCEDURE:　ADMINISTRATION OF INTRAMUSCULAR INJECTIONS

Action	Rationale
Follow steps 1–5 for 'Administration of Subcutaneous Injections'	See steps 1–5 for 'Administration of Subcutaneous Injections'
Clean the chosen site for 30 seconds with alcohol swab and allow the skin to dry for 30 seconds if this is local policy	Reduces pathogens introduced
Stretch the skin, warn the patient and then swiftly insert the needle at 90 degree angle	Facilitates insertion of needle and displaces underlying subcutaneous tissue Ensures needle penetrates muscle
Pull back plunger and if no blood is aspirated, inject the drug slowly. If blood is present, withdraw the needle and reinsert the needle, explaining to the patient	Confirms needle is in the correct position and not in the vein Allows time for the muscle fibres to expand and absorb the solution Prevents pain and ensures an even distribution of drug
Wait for 10 seconds before withdrawing the needle rapidly. Apply pressure to the bleeding point	Allows medication to diffuse into the tissues Prevents haematoma
Refer to steps 9 and 10 of 'Administration of Subcutaneous Injections'	Refer to steps 9 and 10 of 'Administration of Subcutaneous Injections'
Alternatively use Z track technique	Leaves the tissue intact in an indirect line, prevents leakage to the tissue surface, reduces damage to the muscles and reduces deep scars occurring
Do not re-sheath needle and dispose into sharps container	Prevents needle stick injury
Ensure patient comfort and covered. Open door/draw back curtains	Promotes comfort and dignity
Ventrogluteal site cannot be used for children under seven months of age Vastus lateralis site recommended for intramuscular injections for infants under seven months of age	No major blood vessels or nerves here and for infants whose gluteal muscles are poorly developed
Immobilse infant/young child with the parent/guardian consent, assisting	Prevents accidental injury during the administration of the injection
For children dorsogluteal site should not be used for those under three years of age, unless the child is walking for at least a year	Use gluteal muscles which are developed by walking

References

Brooker, C and Waugh, A (2007) *Foundations of Nursing Practice Fundamentals of Holistic Care*. Mosby, Edinburgh.

Dougherty, L and Lister, S (2006) *The Royal Marsden Hospital Manual of Clinical Nursing Procedures*, 6th edn. Blackwell Publishing, Oxford.

Downie, G et al. (2000) Administration of Medicines. In G Downie et al. (eds) *Pharmacology and Drugs Management for Nurses*, 2nd edn. Churchill Livingstone, London.

Greenway, K (2004) Using the Ventrogluteal Site for Intramuscular Injection, *Nursing Standard* 3(18): 39–42.

Greenway, K and Hainsworth, T (2004) Is It Right to be Injecting the Dorsogluteal Site? *Nursing Times Practical Procedure* 100(47): 16.

King, L (2003) Subcutaneous Insulin Injection Technique, *Nursing Standard* 17(34): 45–52.

NMC (2004) *Guidelines for the Administration of Medicines*. NMC, London.

NMC (2005) *Guidelines for Records and Record Keeping*. NMC, London.

NMC (2007) *Guidance for the Introduction of the Essential Skills Clusters for Pre-Registration Nursing Programmes*. NMC, London.

NMC (2008) *The Code Standards of Conduct, Performance and Ethics for Nurses and Midwives*. NMC, London.

Peragollo-Dittko, V (1997) Rethinking Subcutaneous Injection Technique, *American Journal of Nursing* 97(5): 71–72.

Royal College of Paediatrics and Child Health (2002) *Position Statement on Injection Technique*. www.rcph.ac.uk

Weinstein, SM (2007) *Plumer's Principles and Practices of Intravenous Therapy*, 8th edn. Lippincot, Philadelphia.

Workman, B (1999) Safe Injection Techniques, *Nursing Standard* 13(39): 47–53.

12

Wound Care

Learning Outcomes

This chapter is designed to help you:

o   understand the structure of the skin
o   understand wound healing, especially (a) the various stages of the process and (b) the factors that affect healing
o   understand what causes pressure ulcers
o   understand how to prevent pressure sores
o   understand the principles of wound cleaning and wound dressing
o   understand the scope of a nurse's professional responsibilities.

Introduction

The skin is the largest organ of the body. It consists of a number of layers, namely the epidermis; dermis; and subcutaneous layers. The epidermis consists of stratified (i.e., layered) squamous epithelium, where keratin and melanin are found. These protect the skin from harmful substances and from the sun. The epidermis contains no blood vessels or nerve endings. It has hair and contains sweat and sebaceous glands. The epidermis provides a natural barrier against infection: it gradually sheds cells (cells are replaced every 28 days) (Burr and Penzer 2005). Beneath the epidermis is the dermis. The epidermis is connected to the dermis by downward projections (known as rete ridges). These interlock with upward projections (dermal papillae) from the dermis (Powell and Soon 2002).

The dermis is composed of connective tissue and contains blood and lymph vessels, nerve fibres, hair follicles, sweat glands and sebaceous glands. White fibrous tissue and yellow elastic fibres provide toughness and elasticity and also provide the epidermis above with structural and nutritional support (Holloway and Jones 2005).

The subcutaneous tissue is the next layer. This connects the skin to the underlying structures (Williams 2003). Adipose (fat) tissue located here helps to insulate the body from heat and cold.

The skin has a number of functions. It:

- regulates body temperature (through vasodilation and vasoconstriction)
- senses pain, prevents loss of fluid and electrolytes
- prevents micro-organisms from entering the body
- provides protection from harmful effects of ultraviolet light (Williams 2001).

The skin may be damaged by trauma, surgery, incontinence or underlying disease. Skin damage can have both physical and psychological effects upon health and well being. For example, damage may reduce self esteem and make the patient conscious of his or her body image. Thomas-Hess (2000) has suggested a number of practical considerations to maintain skin integrity. These are known as 'Skin Care Basics'.

Box 12.1   Skin Care Basics

Assess the skin at least daily
Clean the skin at frequent intervals with pH balanced cleansing agent, applying moisturisers and barrier cream
Avoid massaging the area concerned and be aware of the force applied that may cause damage
Avoid drying the skin
Position the patient, transfer and turn properly to avoid friction and shearing forces.

(Thomas-Hess 2000)

Skin care planning and wound management requires an holistic assessment (often involving the MDT), informed by an understanding of the normal structure and role of the skin. NMC (2007) specifies that students must be able to 'undertake and document a comprehensive, systematic and accurate nursing assessment'.

Wounds

A wound may be defined as an injury to the body involving a break in the continuity of tissues or of body structures (Martin 2002). Wound care is a broad term relating to managing wounds, preventing tissue damage and care of vulnerable skin. Wounds can occur at any time and age, so a broad understanding of the fundamental principles of wound care is needed to provide a basis for appropriate care. Acute wounds are those that occur suddenly, for example, as a result of surgery, trauma, lacerations or puncturing. Healing may occur over a short period of time. Chronic wounds, in contrast, are those where healing is delayed or interrupted (failing to respond to conservative or surgical treatment). This may result from a longstanding injury, frequent recurrence of an injury, infection, or a coexisting medical condition.

The Healing Process

Wounds can heal by primary, secondary or tertiary intention. Healing involves a series of stages. With changes in skin cell physiology and impairment of the skin's physiological properties, appropriate treatment can prevent further skin damage occurring and induce timely tissue repair (Braiman-Wiksman et al. 2007).

Primary healing occurs where there is minimal tissue loss. It involves drawing the wound edges together with sutures or clips (Miller and Dyson 1996, Dealey 1999). Secondary healing occurs where there is tissue loss and drawing of the edges together is not possible, so the wound is left open, granulates (new tissue is formed) and is used to promote healing. This is the case with pressure sores, for example. However, the open nature of such wounds leaves them susceptible to infections. Tertiary healing or delayed primary closure occurs when an infection or contamination is present in the wound, so healing is delayed until the infection or contamination is removed.

Wound healing is a multi-stage process. The initial stages of wound healing involve the formation of a blood clot and **inflammation**, followed by **proliferation**, the migration of dermal and epidermal cells and matrix synthesis. This process fills the wound gap and re-establishes the skin's barrier (Hackman and Ford 2002, Harding et al. 2005), while tissue remodelling and differentiation enable full recovery of the skin tissue and restore the aesthetics of the skin (Hackman and Ford 2002, Diegelmann and Evans 2004).

The four stages to wound healing are: vascular response (Stage 1); inflammation or inflammatory response (Stage 2); proliferation (Stage 3); and **maturation** (Stage 4) (Miller and Dyson 1996, Calvin 1998, Moore and Foster 1998, Ehrlich 1999, Flanagan 2003).

Stage 1 (0–3 days)   The immediate response is to stop the bleeding and encourage the migration of cells to initiate healing. The blood vessels initially constrict, platelets accumulate at the wound site, stick together (aggregate) and encourage clot formation to form a plug and stop the bleeding. Coagulation factors cause a fibrin clot, where the blood cells are trapped in the fibrin, resulting first in a clot and then a scab or eschar as it dries. This prevents further bleeding and loss of bodily fluids. Damaged cells release histamine, causing the surrounding intact capillaries to dilate and become more permeable. It is this increase in blood flow and leakage of plasma to the tissues that causes local oedema and heat, contributing to the inflamed appearance of the wound.

Stage 2 (1–6 days)   Vasodilation occurs, resulting in gaps between the cells in the capillary walls, and fluid leaks out between the tissues. Extra fluid and an increased blood supply results in redness, heat, swelling and pain with some loss of function and movement. White blood cells are attracted here by protein growth factors to defend against bacteria and remove debris from the wound. Fibroblasts (immature cells forming connective tissue) form collagen which provides a supporting framework in connective tissue. Slough forms, allowing granulation tissue to form in the wound bed, increasing capillary permeability and resulting in exudates from the wound, while an extracellular matrix is formed, thereby allowing new blood vessels to enter. Microbial factors delaying the healing process include infection, increased exudate volume and purulent exudates, toxins from bacteria damage cells, odour, biofilm formation inhibiting healing, slough and necrosis providing an ideal environment for bacterial growth.

Stage 3 (3–20 days)   Fibroblasts are stimulated, multiply and form an extracellular matrix to support new tissue growth. **Angiogenesis** and epithelial cells proliferate and migrate to the wound to facilitate healing and referred-to granulation tissue. The wound then heals by granulation, contraction and **epithelialisation**, whereby fibroblasts form a net-like structure at the wound with granulating tissue; hence the granulation. Collagen fibres are required for shape, prevention of injury and contraction, thereby allowing the wound to shrink in size and develop epithelial tissues (epithelialisation).

Stage 4 (21 days–1 year)   During the final stage of healing the wound appears to be 'healed' because of the layer covering of new skin (epithelial tissue). From the wound edge, sweat glands and hair follicles migrate over the new granulating tissue to complete epithelialisation. Collagen matures, gains strength, exhibits a more orderly structure and new mature blood vessels from capillary dilatation and the number of fibroblasts reduce due to repair rather than regeneration. This leaves the wound healed, with scar tissue forming from fibrous tissue, which initially looks red, slightly raised and itchy, eventually settling. The scar tissue can take up to two years to mature during which time the tissue is remodelling itself with the resulting scar being less elastic and being paler than the surrounding skin.

LEARNING ACTIVITY 12.1

1 When undertaking a dressing and asked to assess a wound, what exactly do you need to assess?
2 What complications may occur?
3 What signs and symptoms might indicate that a wound is infected?

Factors Affecting Wound Healing

The aim of wound management is to ensure the environment is as ideal as possible, in order for healing to occur rapidly. Healing is influenced by a number of factors. A moist environment encourages the migration of the cells carrying out the repair process. The following encourage healing: a diet rich in protein, carbohydrates, lipids, vitamin A and C, iron, zinc (Anderson 2005), optimum blood supply, absence of contaminants, being free from trauma, a healthy immune system, rest and sleep.

Boyd et al. (2004) and Gohel et al. (2005) established a working group to consider the factors that affect wound healing. These they categorised as follows:

- local factors (foreign bodies, incontinence)
- regional factors (oedema, neuropathy, perfusion)
- systemic or patient related factors (age, medication, stress, diabetes, malnutrition, pain, psychological issues).

There are also biological and microbial factors delaying wound healing, though the biological factors were not directly observable. The wound would therefore need to be monitored, assessed and documented if inflammation or infection, moisture, edge or **epithelium** has occurred (Schultz et al. 2003, Gray et al. 2006).

Delayed wound healing can also result from systematic or patient related factors.

Box 12.2   Factors Delaying Wound Healing

Factors Delaying Wound Healing	Rationale
Age	Reduces vascularity, slows cell regeneration, collagen synthesis, poor circulation, thin skin
Poor nutritional status Dehydration	Vitamin C and protein are necessary for collagen synthesis and cell replication
Poor oxygenation	Waste products are retained
Immobility Insulin dependent diabetes mellitus	Pressure on the tissues result in pressure ulcers
Immunosuppressive medication	Affects inflammatory response and immunity
Stress	Cortisol production affects the anti-inflam matory response and may inhibit fibroblasts, collagen synthesis, granulation reducing blood supply
Poor surgical technique Trauma Foreign bodies, e.g., grit, sutures Temperature, e.g., cold	
Medication, e.g., anti-inflammatory drugs	Prevent necessary inflammation of the wound
Poor wound management	Inappropriate dressing inhibits cellular activity
Slough and necrotic tissue	Prevents the healing cascade occurring and inhibits cell migration required for healing-, thereby increasing the risk of infection
Smoking	Reduces the amount of functional haemoglobin in the blood limiting the oxygen carrying capacity of the blood and constricts the arterioles
Nicotine	Impairs macrophages activity, inhibits epithelisation and alters platelet aggregation, thereby increasing thrombus formation

(Whitehead 2003, Dahners and Mullis 2004)

REFER TO PROCEDURE: WOUND MANAGEMENT

LEARNING ACTIVITY 12.2

For your clinical area:

- find out what dressings are available
- identify the functions of each type of dressing
- identify who selects the dressing to be used for a wound.

Pressure Ulcers

Pressure ulcers are localised areas of damage to the skin and underlying tissue caused by pressure, shearing forces, friction, or a combination of the three (Benbow 2006). They can develop in all age groups, all specialities and care settings and can cause distress, pain, embarrassment, increased morbidity, increased care cost and delayed discharge from hospital. Pressure ulcers are classified into four distinct grades – one, two, three and four.

Box 12.3 Pressure Ulcers Classification	
Type	**Appearance**
Grade 1	Skin becomes discoloured, warm, oedematous, hard
Grade 2	Partial thickness of skin, loss of epidermis, dermis or both
	Superficial ulcer appears as an abrasion or blister
Grade 3	Full thickness skin loss with damage to or necrosis of subcutaneous tissue extending to the **fascia**
Grade 4	Extensive damage with tissue necrosis or damage to the muscle, bone or supportin structure, with or without full thickness skin loss
(European Pressure Ulcer Advisory Panel (EPUAP) 1998)	

There are also a number of intrinsic factors that result in pressure ulcer formation. These include age, underlying disease, reduced mobility, poor nutritional status, sensory impairment, incontinence, pain, drugs, reduced consciousness, infection, obesity, malnutrition, dehydration and cognitive and psychological status.

The key to managing pressure ulcers is frequent and systematic assessment in order to ensure that treatment is appropriate and any deterioration is recognised early. EPUAP (1998), NICE (2005) and NPSA (2006) suggest assessments be undertaken daily or at least weekly by a registered healthcare professional to assess, analyse and manage any potential risk and establish any improvement or deterioration, thereby enabling care intervention to be amended accordingly. NICE (2005) recommends guidelines be implemented to prevent pressure ulcer development.

Numerous assessment tools are available for identifying those at risk of developing pressure ulcers. They include the Braden Scale (Bergstrom et al. 1987), Norton Scale (1989) and Waterlow Scale (2005). The tools are based upon assessing who is at risk and the level of risk of developing a pressure sore. They are designed to help nurses to establish the care to be delivered and to measure any improvement or deterioration. Note that there is no substitute for regular assessment.

Note that the way the tools indicate susceptibility to pressure sore development differs. For example, on the Braden Scale the lower the score, the higher the risk of developing a pressure sore, whereas on the Waterlow Scale, the higher the score the greater the risk of developing a pressure sore. The Braden Scale was originally designed to predict the development of pressure ulcers, while the Norton and Waterlow Scales were designed to assess risk more effectively than the nurses' own clinical judgement (Pancorbo-Hidalgo et al. 2006, Waterlow 2005a). The RCN and NICE (2005) advocate the use of tools as an aid to the assessment process, not a replacement for clinical judgements. Therefore, familiarity with whichever assessment tool is used locally is required.

LEARNING ACTIVITY 12.3

- In your area, what assessment tools are used for assessing those at risk of developing a pressure ulcer?
- What are your responsibilities when ensuring that pressure-relieving equipment is in place to reduce pressure (and development of a pressure ulcer)?

Assessment should be made not only of the grade of the pressure ulcer but also of physical and psychological factors; skin condition; cardiovascular and respiratory function; current medication; nutritional status; experience of pain; and any known allergies. Treatment also requires prevention of the development of pressure ulcers. This requires avoidance of friction, pressure and shearing forces, and a consideration of contributory factors such as incontinence. Specialist pressure-relieving equipment such as mattresses, beds, cushions and two hourly repositioning of the patient can help to minimise further development of the ulcer (NICE 2001, Young and Clark 2003). Using moving and handling equipment and prescribed dressings can help to provide an ideal environment for wound healing. Pressure sores and wounds must be reassessed when the patient condition changes (whether through deterioration or improvement) or on transfer to another care setting.

BRADEN SCALE FOR PREDICTING PRESSURE SORE RISK

Patient's Name _____   Evaluator's Name _____   Date of Assessment _____

SENSORY PERCEPTION Ability to respond meaningfully to pressure-related discomfort	**1. Completely Limited** Unresponsive (does not moan, flinch, or grasp) to painful stimuli, due to diminished level of consciousness or sedation OR limited ability to feel pain over most of body	**2. Very Limited** Responds only to painful stimuli. Cannot communicate discomfort except by moaning or restlessness OR has a sensory impairment which limits the ability to feel pain or discomfort over 1/2 of body	**3. Slightly Limited** Responds to verbal commands, but cannot always communicate discomfort or the need to be turned OR has some sensory impairment which limits ability to feel pain or discomfort in 1 or 2 extremities	**4. No Impairment** Responds to verbal commands. Has no sensory deficit which would limit ability to feel or voice pain or discomfort. …			
MOISTURE Degree to which skin is exposed to moisture	**1. Constantly Moist** Skin is kept moist almost constantly by perspiration, urine, etc. Dampness is detected every time patient is moved or turned	**2. Very Moist** Skin is often, but not always moist. Linen must be changed at least once a shift	**3. Occasionally Moist** Skin is occasionally moist, requiring an extra linen change approximately once a day	**4. Rarely Moist** Skin is usually dry, linen only requires changing at routine intervals			
ACTIVITY Degree of physical activity	**1. Bedfast** Confined to bed	**2. Chairfast** Ability to walk severely limited or non-existent. Cannot bear own weight and/or must be assisted into chair or wheelchair	**3. Walks Occasionally** Walks occasionally during day, but for very short distances, with or without assistance. Spends majority of each shift in bed or chair	**4 Walks Frequently** Walks outside room at least twice a day and inside room at least once every two hours during waking hours			
MOBILITY Ability to change and control body position	**1. Completely Immobile** Does not make even slight changes in body or extremity position without assistance	**2. Very Limited** Makes occasional slight changes in body or extremity position but unable to make frequent or significant changes independently	**3. Slightly Limited** Makes frequent though slight changes in body or extremity position independently	**4. No Limitation** Makes major and frequent changes in position without assistance			
NUTRITION Usual food intake pattern	**1. Very Poor** Never eats a complete meal. Rarely eats more than 1/3 of any food offered. Eats 2 servings or less of protein (meat or dairy products) per day. Takes fluids poorly. Does not take a liquid dietary supplement OR is NPO and/or maintained on clear liquids or IVs for more than 5 days	**2. Probably Inadequate** Rarely eats a complete meal and generally eats only about 1/2 of any food offered. Protein intake includes only 3 servings of meat or dairy products per day. Occasionally will take a dietary supplement OR receives less than optimum amount of liquid diet or tube feeding	**3. Adequate** Eats over half of most meals. Eats a total of 4 servings of protein (meat, dairy products) per day. Occasionally will refuse a meal, but will usually take a supplement when offered OR is on a tube feeding or TPN regimen which probably meets most of nutritional needs	**4. Excellent** Eats most of every meal. Never refuses a meal. Usually eats a total of 4 or more servings of meat and dairy products. Occasionally eats between meals. Does not require supplementation			
FRICTION & SHEAR	**1. Problem** Requires moderate to maximum assistance in moving. Complete lifting without sliding against sheets is impossible. Frequently slides down in bed or chair, requiring frequent repositioning with maximum assistance. Spasticity, contractures or agitation leads to almost constant friction	**2. Potential Problem** Moves feebly or requires minimum assistance. During a move skin probably slides to some extent against sheets, chair, restraints or other devices. Maintains relatively good position in chair or bed most of the time but occasionally slides down	**3. No Apparent Problem** Moves in bed and in chair independently and has sufficient muscle strength to lift up completely during move. Maintains good position in bed or chair				

Total Score _____

Source: Barbara Braden and Nancy Bergstrom. Copyright 1988. Reprinted with permission. Permission should be sought to use this tool at www.bradenscale.com

WATERLOW PRESSURE ULCER PREVENTION/TREATMENT POLICY
RING SCORES IN TABLE, ADD TOTAL. MORE THAN 1 SCORE/CATEGORY CAN BE USED

BUILD/WEIGHT FOR HEIGHT	◆	SKIN TYPE VISUAL RISK AREAS	◆	SEX AGE	◆	MALNUTRITION SCREENING TOOL (MST) (Nutrition Vol.15, No.6 1999 - Australia)
AVERAGE BMI = 20-24.9	0	HEALTHY	0	MALE	1	**A - HAS PATIENT LOST WEIGHT RECENTLY**
ABOVE AVERAGE BMI = 25-29.9	1	TISSUE PAPER DRY OEDEMATOUS CLAMMY, PYREXIA	1	FEMALE 14 - 49 50 - 64	2 1 1	YES - GO TO B NO - GO TO C UNSURE - GO TO C AND SCORE 2
OBESE BMI > 30	2	DISCOLOURED GRADE 1	2	65 - 74	2	**B - WEIGHT LOSS SCORE** 0.5 - 5kg = 1; 5 - 10kg = 2; 10 - 15kg = 3; >15kg = 4; unsure = 2
BELOW AVERAGE BMI < 20 BMI=Wt(Kg)/Ht (m)²	3	BROKEN/SPOTS GRADE 2-4	3	75 - 80 81 +	4 5	**C - PATIENT EATING POORLY OR LACK OF APPETITE** 'NO' = 0; 'YES' SCORE = 1; **NUTRITION SCORE** If > 2 refer for nutrition assessment / intervention

CONTINENCE	◆	MOBILITY	◆	TISSUE MALNUTRITION	◆	NEUROLOGICAL DEFICIT	◆
COMPLETE/ CATHETERISED	0	FULLY	0	TERMINAL CACHEXIA	8	DIABETES, MS, CVA	4-6
URINE INCONT.	1	RESTLESS/FIDGETY	1	MULTIPLE ORGAN FAILURE	8	MOTOR/SENSORY	4-6
FAECAL INCONT.	2	APATHETIC	2	SINGLE ORGAN FAILURE (RESP, RENAL, CARDIAC,)	5	PARAPLEGIA (MAX OF 6)	4-6
URINARY + FAECAL INCONTINENCE	3	RESTRICTED BEDBOUND e.g. TRACTION CHAIRBOUND e.g. WHEELCHAIR	3 4 5	PERIPHERAL VASCULAR DISEASE ANAEMIA (Hb < 8) SMOKING	5 2 1	**MAJOR SURGERY or TRAUMA** ORTHOPAEDIC/SPINAL 5; ON TABLE > 2 HR# 5; ON TABLE > 6 HR# 8	

SPECIAL RISKS

MEDICATION - CYTOTOXICS, LONG TERM/HIGH DOSE STEROIDS, ANTI-INFLAMMATORY MAX OF 4

SCORE	
10+ AT RISK	
15+ HIGH RISK	
20+ VERY HIGH RISK	

Scores can be discounted after 48 hours provided patient is recovering normally

© J Waterlow 1985 Revised 2005*
Obtainable from the Nook, Stoke Road, Henlade TAUNTON TA3 5LX
* The 2005 revision incorporates the research undertaken by Queensland Health.

www.judy-waterlow.co.uk

Source: Printed with permission of Judy Waterlow SRN RCNT www.judy-waterlow.co.uk

REMEMBER TISSUE DAMAGE MAY START PRIOR TO ADMISSION, IN CASUALTY. A SEATED PATIENT IS AT RISK
ASSESSMENT (See Over) IF THE PATIENT FALLS INTO ANY OF THE RISK CATEGORIES, THEN PREVENTATIVE NURSING IS
REQUIRED A COMBINATION OF GOOD NURSING TECHNIQUES AND PREVENTATIVE AIDS WILL BE NECESSARY
ALL ACTIONS MUST BE DOCUMENTED

PREVENTION
PRESSURE REDUCING AIDS
Special Mattress/beds:
10+ Overlays or specialist foam mattresses.
15+ Alternating pressure overlays, mattresses and bed systems
20+ Bed systems: Fluidised bead, low air loss and alternating pressure mattresses
Note: Preventative aids cover a wide spectrum of specialist features. Efficacy should be judged, if possible, on the basis of independent evidence.
No person should sit in a wheelchair without some form of cushioning. If nothing else is available – use the person's own pillow. (Consider infection risk)

Cushions:
10+ 100mm foam cushion
15+ Specialist Gell and/or foam cushion
20+ Specialised cushion, adjustable to individual person.

Bed clothing:
Avoid plastic draw sheets, inco pads and tightly tucked in sheet/sheet covers, especially when using specialist bed and mattress overlay systems
Use duvet - plus vapour permeable membrane.

NURSING CARE
General
HAND WASHING, frequent changes of position, lying, sitting. Use of pillows
Pain
Appropriate pain control
Nutrition
High protein, vitamins and minerals
Patient Handling
Correct lifting technique - hoists - monkey poles
Transfer devices
Patient Comfort Aids
Real Sheepskin - bed cradle
Operating Table
Theatre/A&E Trolley
100mm(4ins) cover plus adequate protection

Skin Care
General hygiene, NO rubbing, cover with an appropriate dressing

WOUND GUIDELINES
Assessment
odour, exudate, measure/photograph position

WOUND CLASSIFICATION - EPUAP
GRADE 1
Discolouration of intact skin not affected by light finger pressure (non-blanching erythema)
This may be difficult to identify in darkly pigmented skin

GRADE 2
Partial thickness skin loss or damage involving epidermis and/or dermis
The pressure ulcer is superficial and presents clinically as an abrasion, blister or shallow crater

GRADE 3
Full thickness skin loss involving damage of subcutaneous tissue but not extending to the underlying fascia.
The pressure ulcer presents clinically as a deep crater with or without undermining of adjacent tissue

GRADE 4
Full thickness skin loss with extensive destruction and necrosis extending to underlying tissue.

Dressing Guide
Use Local dressings formulary and/or www.worldwidewounds

IF TREATMENT IS REQUIRED, FIRST REMOVE PRESSURE

Source: Printed with permission of Judy Waterlow SRN RCNT. www.judy-waterlow.co.uk

REFER TO PROCEDURE: PREVENTING PRESSURE ULCER FORMATION

Principles of Wound Cleaning

The aim of wound cleaning is to create an optimum local environment for healing to occur by removing debris, exudate, foreign and necrotic material, toxic components, bacteria and other micro-organisms. In order to achieve this the following need to be assessed – cause, location, size and shape of the wound, characteristics of the wound bed (in open wounds) and margin, degree of exudate, presence of infection, odour from the wound, pain, condition of the surrounding skin, any other complications present (e.g., haematuria), presence of foreign bodies, type of skin closure, drains, previous wound and dressings used. Preventing a wound forming requires a multidisciplinary team approach that includes a risk assessment, working with the patient, and drawing on the expertise of a tissue viability nurse, doctor, dietician and pharmacist.

The wound should be free from infection and cleaned using an aseptic technique (refer to Procedure: Aseptic Technique). If superficial slough, pus, excessive exudate or visible debris is present, clean the wound with saline as it does not have a toxic effect on the skin. It also removes particulate matter, surface bacteria and remnants of the dressings without damaging cells or delaying healing. Sodium chloride (0.9 per cent) is a physiologically balanced solution compatible with the body. It is the safest and most appropriate cleaning solution for non-contaminated solutions (Miller and Dyson 1996, Fletcher 1997). It does not have any antiseptic properties but does dilute bacteria and is non-toxic to tissue (Morgan 2000).

Cotton wool balls or gauze may shed fibres, causing inflammation and therefore delaying wound healing as a warm, moist environment is required. Rather than use either of these, irrigate the wound instead. Cleansing may cool the wound. The surrounding skin should be cleaned to remove the dressing material or exudate, which is detrimental to the skin and wound, as it can result in the skin and wound breaking down. Instead of cleaning the wound routinely or on a daily basis, any decision made to clean the wound should be made on an individual basis with the tissue viability nurse and medical team.

REFER TO PROCEDURE: WOUND MANAGEMENT

Wound Dressings

The selection of dressing will depend on the condition of the wound site and surrounding skin, the patient's needs, wishes and lifestyle, cost effectiveness and product availability. Wound dressings may be either passive or interactive dressings. Passive dressings protect against physical damage and should only be used for healed surgical wounds and superficial wounds: they do not have the characteristics of an ideal dressing. Interactive dressings maximise healing by sealing off the wound from the environment: they are semi-permeable or impermeable to water vapour and micro-organisms.

Decision Tree for Wound Management

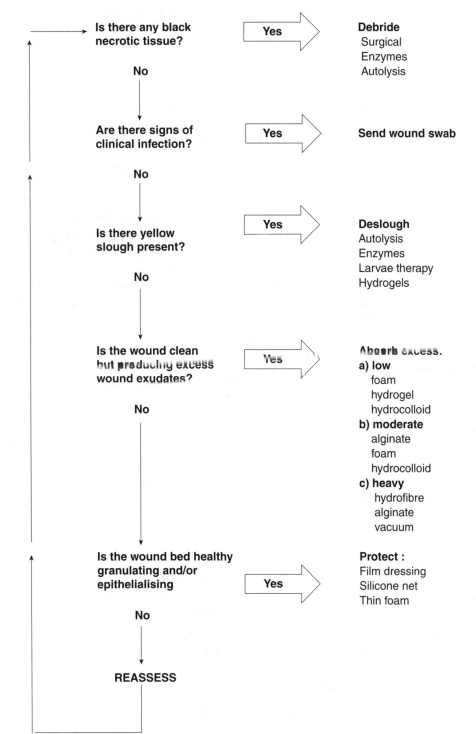

Is there any black necrotic tissue? → **Yes** → **Debride**
Surgical
Enzymes
Autolysis

No

Are there signs of clinical infection? → **Yes** → **Send wound swab**

No

Is there yellow slough present? → **Yes** → **Deslough**
Autolysis
Enzymes
Larvae therapy
Hydrogels

No

Is the wound clean but producing excess wound exudates? → **Yes** → **Absorb excess.**
a) **low**
foam
hydrogel
hydrocolloid
b) **moderate**
alginate
foam
hydrocolloid
c) **heavy**
hydrofibre
alginate
vacuum

No

Is the wound bed healthy granulating and/or epithelialising → **Yes** → **Protect :**
Film dressing
Silicone net
Thin foam

No

REASSESS

The ideal dressing is one that has the following characteristics – it maintains a moist wound site, provides thermal insulation, provides a barrier to micro-organisms (to and from the wound), protects the wound from trauma, is toxic and non-allergenic, allows gaseous exchange, is sterile, won't shred fibres into the wound, is flexible, comfortable, conforming, available, controls odour and exudate, is acceptable to the patient, requires infrequent changing, is cost effective and has a reasonable shelf life and storage requirement.

For dry, black necrotic wounds debride and rehydrate the wound, while for yellow, sloughy wounds, remove the slough by debriding and cleaning. For red, granulating wounds protect and maintain the moisture balance with enough exudate to keep the wound moist and promote cell movement, while for pink epithelialising wounds protect and maintain the moisture.

Professional Responsibilities

Nurses have a professional responsibility to recognise the limitations of their own expertise, maintain their professional development and keep abreast of changes within practice. This requirement certainly applies to wound care and use of dressings. This corresponds with the NMC (2008) who state that 'you must recognise and work within the limits of your competence' and 'you must deliver care based on the best available evidence or best practice'. This requires an awareness not only of cleaning solutions and the range of dressings used, but also of a wide range of other factors. They include referrals made to and advice sought from the tissue viability nurse, health education and health promotion, teaching, standards of care development, benchmarking, guidelines, protocols, procedures, policies, auditing, documentation and nurse-led clinics. Patient and family involvement are also important as they facilitate compliance with treatment and cooperation.

Summary

An holistic approach to wound care and management is required to supporting patients with wounds. This may require interdisciplinary working. Ongoing education and use of evidence-based care is also required to maintain professional knowledge and understanding of the types of wounds, the physiology of wound healing and wound assessment.

PROCEDURE: WOUND MANAGEMENT	
Action	Rationale
Explain and discuss the procedure with the patient Obtain consent	Ensures patient understanding and any consent is informed and valid
Wash and dry hands thoroughly Clean dressing trolley	Prevents cross-infection Provides for a clean work surface

Place all equipment required on bottom shelf of cleaned trolley	Keep top shelf as a clean work surface area
Wear apron and take trolley to patient, disturbing environment as little as possible	Reduces risk of cross-infection Minimises air bourne contamination
Position patient comfortably in area where dressing to be undertaken and do not expose unduly	Maintains patient privacy, dignity, comfort Allows air bourne organisms to settle before sterile field is exposed
Close doors/draw curtains Adjust bed to correct height	Prevents stooping and bending
Clean hands with alcohol hand rub Check dressing pack and all other equipment intact and sterile. If not, discard If sterile, open packaging and slide contents on to top shelf touching only corners and arrange sterile field	Prevents risk of cross-infection Ensures only sterile products used Ensures area for potential contamination are kept to a minimum Prevents environmental contamination and minimises risk of contamination of cleaning solution
Where appropriate, loosen old dressing, remove and clean hands with alcohol hand rub	Dressing can be removed without causing trauma To reduce the risk of wound infection having removed the dressing Prevents cross infection
Attach bag to side of dressing trolley below top shelf	Ensures contaminated material below level of sterile field
While applying gloves assess wound for healing, granulated tissue, epithelialisation and any signs of infection	Reduces risk of infection to the wound and contamination of nurse Evaluate wound care and wound itself Gloves cause less trauma to the wound and skin
Gently clean or irrigate the wound with prescribed solution. Normasol sufficient	Reduces possibility of physical and chemical trauma to granulation and epithelial tissue
Apply prescribed dressing to the wound Fasten dressing with tape or bandage or retention dressing	Promotes healing and reduces symptoms Prevents skin irritation and avoids trauma to the wound
Ensure patient is comfortable and dressing is secure	Dressing may slip or feels uncomfortable as patient changes position
Dispose of waste and gloves into yellow plastic bag	Prevents environmental contamination and waste is incinerated
Draw curtains back/open door/window Ensure patient is comfortable, environment meets patient needs and readjust bed to lower height	Ensures patient has everything to hand and can be independent and self caring Prevents patient falling out of bed

(Cont'd)

Action	Rationale
Clean trolley with chlorhexidine and paper towels Wash and dry hands thoroughly according to local policy	Reduces risk of infection
Document the care given	Accurate record keeping and effective communication

PROCEDURE: PREVENTING PRESSURE ULCER FORMATION

Action	Rationale
Assess patient on admission using appropriate tool, e.g., Braden Scale, Waterlow Scale	Identifies patient at risk of developing pressure ulcer
Reassess patient regularly and whether there has been a deterioration or improvement in their condition	Provides data and information on which to base treatment upon
Do not rub area at risk	Rubbing causes maceration and degeneration of subcutaneous tissue, especially in the elderly
Wash area at risk if patient incontinent or sweating profusely, using mild soap (if they allow). Rinse and dry thoroughly, using moisturiser if skin very dry. Ask what patient prefers	Maintains skin integrity Prevents ulcer forming Gentle drying promotes comfort and discourages micro-organisms' growth Cracked dry skin allows micro-organisms to enter
Barrier creams used as indicated and prescribed	Barrier creams prevent damage to the epidermis but are occlusive and prevent exchange from the skin
Educate and encourage repositioning Examine vulnerable areas regularly, e.g., two hourly	Encourages patient participation in care
Mobilise patient in conjunction with therapists, e.g., physiotherapist	Reduces further tissue damage and improves circulation
Use pressure-relieving devices, e.g., mattresses, chairs, two hourly turns	Reduces pressure where possible
Have patient recumbent where possible Support with pillows in bed Reduce period sitting in chair	Avoid bed rests as they increase shearing by allowing patient to slide down the bed

References

Anderson, B (2005) Nutrition and Wound Healing: The Necessity of Assessment, *British Journal of Nursing* 14(19 Suppl): S30, S32, S34, S36, S38.

Bergstrom, N et al. (1987) The Braden Scale for Predicting Pressure Sore Risk, *Nursing Research* 36(4): 205–210.

Benbow, M (2006) An Update on VAC Therapy, *Journal of Community Nursing* 4(11): 647–651.

Boyd, C et al. (2004) Prevention of Non-Healing Wounds Through the Prediction of Chronicity, *Journal of Wound Care* 13(7): 265–266.

Braiman-Wiksman, L et al. (2007) Novel Insights into Wound Healing Sequence of Events, *Toxicologic Pathology* 35: 767–779.

Burr, S and Penzer, R (2005) Promoting Skin Care, *Nursing Standard* 19(36): 57–65.

Calvin, M (1998) Cutaneous Wound Repair, *Wounds* 10(1): 12–32.

Dahners, LE and Mullis, BH (2004) Effect of Non-Steroidal Anti-Inflammatory Drugs on Bone Formation and Soft tissue, *Healing Journal of American Academic Orthopaedic Surgery* 12(3): 130–143.

Dealey, C (1999) *The Care of Wounds: A Guide for Nurses*, 2nd edn. Blackwell Science, Oxford.

Diegelmann, RF and Evans, MC (2004) Wound Healing: An Overview of Acute, Fibrotic and Delayed Healing Front, *Biosci* 9: 283–289.

Ehrlich, HP (1999) The Physiology of Wound Healing: A Summary of Normal and Abnormal Wound Healing Processes, *Advanced Wound Care* 11(7): 326–328.

European Pressure Ulcer Advisory Panel (1998) *Pressure Ulcer Treatment Guidelines*. www.epuap.org/gltreatment.html

Flanagan, M (2003) Wound Management: Can it Help us to Monitor Progression to Healing? *Journal of Wound Care* 12(5): 189–194.

Fletcher, J (1997) Update: Wound Cleaning, *Professional Nurse* 12(11): 793–796.

Gohel, MS et al. (2005) Risk Factors for Delayed Wound Healing and Recurrence of Chronic Venous Leg Ulcers – An Analysis of 1324 Legs, *European Journal of Vascular and Endovascular Surgery* 29(1): 74–77.

Gray, D et al. (2006) A Clinical Audit of a Tissue Viability Service Using Applied Wound Management, *Wounds UK* 2(2): 47–59.

Hackman, DJ and Ford, HR (2002) Cellular, Biochemical and Clinical Aspects of Wound Healing, *Surgical Infect* 3(Suppl 1): S23–S25.

Harding, KG et al. (2005) Wound Chrinicity and Fibroblast Senescence – Implications for Treatment, *International Wound Journal* 2: 364–368.

Holloway, S and Jones, V (2005) The Importance of Skin Care and Assessment, *British Journal of Nursing* 14(22): 1172–1176.

Martin, EA (2002) *Concise Colour Medical Dictionary*. Oxford University Press, Oxford.

Miller, M and Dyson, M (1996) *Principles of Wound Care*. Macmillan, London.

Morgan, DA (2000) *Formulary of Wound Management Products: A Guide for Healthcare Staff*, 8th edn. (Internet Update). Euromed Communications, Haslemere.

Moore, P and Foster, L (1998) Acute Surgical Wound Care 2: The Wound Healing Process, *British Journal of Nursing* 7(19): 1183–1187.

NICE (2001) *Pressure Ulcer Risk: Assessment and Prevention*. NICE, London.

NICE (2005) *CG29 Pressure Ulcer Management: Quick Reference Guide*. www.guidance.nice.org.uk

NMC (2007) *Guidance for the Introduction of the Essential Skills Clusters for Pre-Registration Nursing Programmes*. NMC, London.

NMC (2008) *The Code: Standards of Conduct, Performance and Ethics for Nurses and Midwives*. NMC, London.

Norton, D (1989) Calculating the Risk Reflections on the Norton Scale, *Decubitus* 20(3): 24–31.

NPSA (2006) *Risk Assessment Programme: Overview*. www.npsa.nhs.uk

Pancorbo-Hidalgo, PL et al. (2006) Risk Assessment Scales 4 Pressure Ulcer Prevention: A Systematic Review, *Journal of Advanced Nursing* 54(1): 94–110.

Powell, J and Soon, C (2002) Physiology of the Skin, *Surgery* 20(6): ii–vi.

RCN and NICE (2005) *Management of Pressure Ulcers in Primary and Secondary Care A Clinical Practice Guidance*. www.rcn.org.uk/publications

Schultz, GS et al. (2003) Wound Bed Preparation: A Systematic Approach to Wound Management, *Wound Repair and Regeneration 11 Supplement 1*: S1–S28.

Thomas-Hess, C (2000) Skin Care Basics, *Advanced Skin Wound Care* 13(3): 127–128.

Waterlow, J (2005) *Pressure Ulcer Prevention Manual*. Waterlow, Taunton.

Waterlow, J (2005a) From Costly Treatment to Cost Effective Prevention: Using Waterlow, *Wound Care* 10 (9 Suppl): 525–530.

Whitehead, L (2003) Nicotine, CO and HCN: The Detrimental Effects of Smoking on Wound Healing, *British Journal of Community Nursing* 8(12 Suppl): S22–S26.

Williams, C (2001) 3M Cavilon Durabel Barrier Cream in Skin Problem Management, *British Journal of Nursing* 10(7): 469–472.

Williams, AC (2003) Structure and Function of Human Skin. In *Transdermal and Topical Drug Delivery: From Theory to Clinical Practice*. Pharmaceutical, London.

Young, T and Clark, M (2003) *Re-Positioning for Pressure Ulcer Prevention (Protocol)*. The Cochrane Library, Wrexham, Wales.

www.smtl.co.uk

www.smtl.co.uk/world–wide–wounds

Answer Guide

Chapter 3

Learning Activity 3.1

Options include:

- Contacting an interpreter and communicating through them
- Communicating through a mixture of verbal and non-verbal signs
- Involve the family.

Learning Activity 3.2

Recommendations include discussion with your mentor, psychiatrist, CPN, family, reminiscence therapy, music, art therapy.

Learning Activity 3.4

Recommended action: speak to the psychiatrist, arrange a meeting so all views can be expressed and reassure the client that ECT is a recognised intervention in mental health.

Learning Activity 3.6

a) Data protection, illegal access
b) Information continuously changing
c) Never being updated.

Learning Activity 3.8

a) Breach of confidentiality
b) Not conveying any information, refusing to confirm any information.

Reflection 1

Physical – nutrition/dehydration; bowels (constipation); infection; side effects of drugs; TIA's; diabetes; thyroid problem.

Psychological – grief/bereavement; depression; anxiety; dementia.

Social – loneliness/isolation; lack of stimulation; neighbours perception of the situation; cultural differences.

Environmental – carbon monoxide poisoning.

Spiritual – questioning his belief in God; frightened about his sense of self.

Reflection 2

Physical – rheumatoid arthritis; chronic pain.

Psychological – stress; effects of hospitalisation and level of dependency; loss of wife as main carer; altered body image.

Professional – choice; informed consent; advocacy and empowerment; duty of care; values and attitudes of staff; partnership in care.

Social – illness behaviour; role change; expert patient.

Nursing – moving and handling assessment and safe practice; immobility (skin integrity); dealing with aggression; privacy and dignity; communication.

Reflection 3

Pathophysiology – knowledge of the skeleton; simple classification of fractures and healing; vital signs in children.

Professional – consent in children; advocacy and empowerment; family centre care, partnership with the family.

Nursing – moving and handling; immobility; skin integrity; skin traction; privacy and dignity; meeting hygiene and elimination needs; communicating with children and their family; pain recognition, assessment and management.

Psychology – effects of stress and hospitalisation on children and their family; effects of accident; loss of control of parents, roles; change or routine and implications; cognitive development.

Sociology – family structure; family life cycle; gender roles; role disruption; impact of missing school, friends; socialisation and development.

Chapter 4

Learning Activity 4.1

1) A micro-organism is any organism not visible to the unaided eye
2) Examples include:

- Bacteria – staphylococcus (MRSA), streptococcus, salmonella
- Virus – meningitis, polio, herpes, measles
- Fungi – candida albicans (thrush), chlamydia.

Learning Activity 4.2

Factors include: extremes of age; underlying disease (AIDS, diabetes, vascular disease); invasive devices (IV and epidural lines, urinary catheters, PEG tubes); surgery; invasive procedures (intubation, endoscopy); drug therapy; known communicable disease (TB); diarrhoea and vomiting.

Learning Activity 4.5

Note that employees should always wear gloves when handling dirty or contaminated laundry and all dirty laundry bags should be collected in a designated laundry container only. Once the laundry is disposed of in the laundry room, employees should wash their hands, having removed the gloves. The clean linen should be delivered either before or after all the dirty linen bags are collected so there is no potential cross-infection.

Learning Activity 4.6

a) Factors include age; home circumstances; admission diagnosis; mobility; diarrhoea and vomiting.
b) Protective clothing to be worn includes fluid repellent footwear; face mask; gloves; and apron.

Chapter 5

Learning Activity 5.2

No, it is not appropriate. Keeping the ward cool is not only important for patient and staff comfort, but reduces the number of bacteria on the ward. However, integrity of the sterile field should never be compromised and airflow should be minimised when doing a dressing. Ceiling fans or open windows are only acceptable if fans are kept clean, blades wiped frequently, windows have intact, meshed screens and can be opened from the top. If opening a window is necessary, rearrange or remove some of the furnishings so a sterile trolley is not near the window or fan.

Chapter 6

Learning Activity 6.1

Oral, Axilla, Rectum

Advantages: easy access; good blood supply; well insulated from external environmental influences on the temperature; easy to use; low cost.

Disadvantages: not used for newborns or children, epileptics, confused or agitated individuals; unreliable in detecting hypothermia; lacks sensitivity in raised body temperature; time taken to record the temperature (2–3 minutes orally, 3–6 minutes axilla and rectum); risk of cross-infection; lack of accuracy.

Tympanic

Advantages: accurate and reliable; good blood supply; fast measurement; easy to use.

Disadvantages: expensive; affected by the ambient temperature; hearing aids have to be removed before use; earwax, blood, foreign bodies in the ear canal can reduce the temperature.

Critical Reflection

Place Mr Kellor on supplementary oxygen due to the low saturation level and cyanosis and inform your mentor/medical team.

Reassure Mr Kellor.

Mrs James's symptoms are classic signs of hypovolaemia caused by fluid loss so inform mentor/medical team for fluids to be replaced.

Reassure Mrs James.

Learning Activity 6.2

Adult – oral, axilla, tympanic (latter especially if patient confused, agitated or disorientated).

Child/Mental Health – axilla, tympanic.

1 Aphasia/dysphagia; ET in situ; language barrier; alcohol; medication; facial/oral injury; hearing impairment; shyness (in children).
2 Stage of development; verbal understanding and ability; trust/reluctance to participate with strangers.
3 Noise; environment; knowledge of child development; time; location; knowledge of the Glasgow Coma Scale; assessment; previous impairment; disease; cooperation of patient/relative/carer intervention.
4 Stress; lack of exercise; excessive alcohol intake; side effects of drugs; age; smoking; caffeine; disease (diabetes, renal failure).
5 Anxiety; exercise; hot drinks/heavy meals; lying versus standing; time of day; noise; equipment used.
6 Pregnancy; exercise; sleep; age; anxiety/stress; infection; heart/lung disease; lack of oxygen; pain; haemorrhage.
7 Age; temperature; pain; level of consciousness; underlying disease, e.g., heart/lung disease, asthma.
8 Time of day; method used to record temperature; presence of disease/infection/inflammation; accuracy in recording; drinks; smoking.
9 Dependent upon age of the child and if able to tolerate oral thermometer. Commonly, tympanic or axilla temperature taken if child held on a lap and arms around the child.
10 Infection; neurological injury; heat exhaustion; reaction to drugs.
11 Immobility; malnutrition; drugs/alcohol; poverty; exposure.
12 The hypothalamus.
13 35.6–37.8 degrees celcius.

Chapter 7

Learning Activity 7.4

1) Visually by looking in Alex's mouth with a pen torch light
2) Pen torch, oral care plan (e.g., by Sarah Freer)
3) Documenting in the care plan, re-evaluating the mouth and asking Alex how his mouth feels.

Chapter 8

Learning Activity 8.1

Underlying issues include lack of respect, dignity, religious needs and family's request not being met; failure to provide correct food; lack of understanding by the nurses; potential breach of Human Rights; and the incident could be reported if witnessed by another individual.

Learning Activity 8.2

Hold a meeting with the multidisciplinary team, John and his mother to discuss the concerns and to agree a plan of care.

Chapter 9

Learning Activity 9.1

- Poor practice
- Poor standards
- Poor communication
- Lack of care
- Possible neglect
- Lack of dignity and respect
- Patient/practitioner expectation of care differing
- Improve all of the above

Chapter 10

Learning Activity 10.2

Quietly leave the room and return 20 minutes later to offer the medication again, as Alzheimer sufferers have periods of irritability and short term memory loss. After a cooling down period sufferers can become compliant, so if the nurse adopts a calm, friendly approach Mrs Gant is likely to comply.

Learning Activity 10.3

Do not leave the antibiotics on the locker. Ask Joanne to either take them there and then or give them to her directly on her return from the toilet.

Chapter 11

Learning Activity 11.1

Stop her colleague from giving the injection and from providing patient care; inform the ward manager and ask for replacement staff, documenting the incident. The Code is jeopardising safety and should be removed. The public expects nurses to be capable of carrying out their duties competently, physically and mentally. The inability to landmark means safety standards have been violated.

Learning Activity 11.2

1) Explain the reason for the injection; use a toy to demonstrate the injection won't hurt
2) Topical or oral administration. Possibly use emla cream.

Learning Activity 11.3

Ask Gavin to repeat what he has been told/understands; write down information; repeat explanations; document in social care plan; refer to the prescription.

Drug Calculations

1) 1.2 mls
2) 1.5 mls
3) 41.5 or 42 drops/min
4) 4
5) 600mg/dose
6) 45 drops/min
7) 1.25 mls
8) 10 mls
9) 20 mls
10) 30mg/dose.

Chapter 12

Learning Activity 12.1

1) Factors to be assessed include size; colour; odours; the skin around the wound; whether dressing is appropriate; whether the wound is healing

2) Necrosis
3) Signs and symptoms of infection include redness; inflammation; pyrexia; odour; the wound is hot to touch; sloughing.

Learning Activity 12.2

Classes of wound dressings and their functions.

Dressing Classification	Main Functions	Examples
Absorbent	Absorb light–heavy exudate	Mesorb
Alginates	Absorption of exudate Haemostasis	Sorbsan, Kaltostat
Antibacterial cream/gel	Odour control and treatment for infection	Flamazine, Metrotop gel
Antimicrobial silver impregnated	Clinically infected	Actisorb sliver
Biological	Debridement	Larva therapy
Cavity	Medium/heavy absorption	Sorbsan ribbon, Allevyn cavity
Deodorising	Odour control	Carboflex
Enzymes	Debridement	Varidase
Foams	Absorption/protection	Lyofoam, Tielle
Hydrocolloids	Absorption/debridement/ protection	Comfeel, Duoderm
Hydrofibres	Absorption	Aquacel
Hydrogels	Debridement	Intrasite
Iodine impregnated	Clinically infected	Inadine, Iodoflex
Low-adherent	Protection	N–A Ultra
Non-adherent silicone	Protection	Mepitel
Paraffin gauze	Protection	Paratulle
Paste impregnated bandages	Skin conditions associated with leg ulcers	Zipzoc, Steripaste
Protese modulating matrix	Rebalancing the pathological wound environment	Promogran
Vapour permeable	Protection/maintaining moist environment	Opsite

Glossary

Adrenaline   a hormone and neurotransmitter. It increases the 'fight or flight' response of the sympathetic division of the autonomic nervous system.

Adipose tissue   specialised connective tissue storage site for fat cushioning and insulating the body.

Aggression   hostile or destructive attitude to other people or objects, which can include verbal attacks or physical violence.

Aldosterone   hormone secreted by the adrenal cortex controlling salt and water in the body.

Angiogenesis   development of new blood vessels resulting in vascularisation of a tissue. This normally occurs after an injury and is part of the repair mechanism.

Anti-diuretic hormone (ADH) a hormone which regulates water retention when dehydrated, causing the kidneys to conserve water but not salt by concentrating the urine and reducing urine volume.

Anti-pyretics   medication used to reduce temperature.

Arrhythmia   variation from the normal rhythm of the heart beat.

Asepsis   absence of micro-organisms.

Auditory   sense of hearing.

Auscultation   listening to internal organs using a stethoscope.

Autonomic nervous system (ANS)   regulatory activity of the smooth and cardiac muscles and glands. It is involuntary in its action and divided into the parasympathetic and sympathetic branches.

Bacteria   unicellular micro-organisms, some of which can cause disease.

Buccal   relating to the cheek.

Bradycardia   slow heart beat slowing the pulse rate to less than 60 beats per minute.

Catheter   tube inserted into the body to introduce or remove fluid.

Cerebral herniation   displacement of brain tissue, cerebrospinal fluid and blood vessels outside the compartments in the head they normally occupy.

Chemoreceptors   receptors sensitive to chemical changes in the bloodstream.

Cushing's triad (reflex)   triad of hypertension, bradycardia and irregular respirations. It is a sign of raised intracranial pressure, cerebral haemorrhage, brain tumour or cerebal herniation.

Cytostatic   an agent that inhibits or suppresses cellular growth and multiplication.

Cytotoxic   chemicals that are directly toxic to cells preventing reproduction or growth.

Dehydration   a condition due to excessive loss of body fluid.

Dermis   layer beneath the epidermis.

Diaphragm   sheet of muscle separating the thorax and abdomen.

Diastolic pressure   resting period in the cardiac cycle. Pressure exerted on the arterial walls represented as the lower value of a blood pressure reading.

Duty of care   a legal or moral obligation that a person has to perform actions for another's welfare.

Encopresis   voluntary or involuntary passing of faeces after bowel control has been achieved in the absence of a known cause.

Enteral feeding   meeting daily nutritional requirements in liquid form through direct insertion into the stomach or small intestine via a tube.

Epidermis   external, non-vascular layer of the skin.

Epinephrine   hormone carried in the blood and a neurotransmitter when released across the neuronal synapse.

Epithelialisation   growth of epithelium over a wound, final stage of wound healing process.

Epithelium   tissue composed of a layer of cells.

Fascia   flat layers of fibrous tissue that separate different layers of tissue.

Fibrillation   rapid and irregular contraction of the heart.

Fungi   organisms that lack chlorophyll and live as parasites.

Hazard   an event or situation that has the potential to cause harm.

Heart rate   frequency of the cardiac cycle calculated as the number of contractions (heart rate) of the heart in one minute and expressed as beats per minute.

Homeostasis   physiological process of maintaining a stable, internal environment.

Hygiene   bodily cleanliness that promotes health and well being.

Hyperaesthesia   neurologic symptom where there is an unusual increase or altered sensitivity to sensory stimuli.

Hypertension   abnormally high blood pressure.

Hyperventilation   excessively hard and fast breathing resulting in too much oxygen in the body.

Hypoaesthesia   partial loss of sensation.

Hypotension   abnormally low blood pressure.

Hypothalamus   small cone-shaped structure in the brain regulating thirst, hunger, temperature, water balance, blood pressure.

Hypothermia   low body temperature.

Hypoventilation   shallow or slow breathing resulting in reduced air entry into the lungs.

Hypovolaemia   low blood volume.

Hyperthermia (pyrexia)   abnormally high body temperature.

Hypoxia   reduced oxygen on the blood.

Infection   an invasion of the body by pathogenic micro-organisms or the result of disease.

Inflammation   the body's self protective reaction to infection or injury.

Malnutrition   a disorder of nutrition.

Maturation process of maturing.

Medulla oblongata lower portion of the brainstem controlling autonomic functions and relaying nerve signals between the brain and spinal cord.

Micro-organism an organism of microscopic size which may or may not cause a disease.

Near miss act or omission that could have led to unintended or unexpected harm, loss or damage but did not actually do so.

Necrosis death of tissue as a result of ischaemia, disease process or failure of blood supply.

Negligence civil wrong where the defendant has breached duty of care and caused some injury, loss or damage to the claimant, of a type the law acknowledges.

Non-verbal communication communication by way of facial expression, gesture, posture, tone of voice, accent.

Norepinephrine released from the adrenal medulla of the adrenal glands as a hormone into the blood. A neurotransmitter in the central nervous system and sympathetic nervous system.

Nosocomial infection an infection acquired or occurring in hospital.

Palpation physical examination by pressing on the surface of the body to feel the organs or tissue underneath.

Parasympathetic nervous system division of the autonomic nervous system that slows heart rate, increases intestinal and gland activity, relaxes sphincter muscles and works with the sympathetic nervous system.

Parenteral nutrition a method of feeding that bypasses the gastrointestinal tract and administers a slow infusion of nutrients directly into the veins.

Pharmacodynamics study of biochemical and physiological effects of drugs and mechanisms of their actions.

Pharmacokinetics a study of the action of drugs in the body and the way in which the body metabolises a drug.

Pons lies between the medulla and cerebellum, appearing as a broad band of transverse fibres.

Proliferation growth or production of cells, rapid and often excessive spread or increase of cells.

Pyrexia   abnormally high body temperature.

Reticular-activating system (RAS)   part of brain maintaining consciousness located in the centre of the brainstem between the medulla oblongata and midbrain.

Risk   anything that has the potential to cause harm.

Risk assessment   assessing the probability of a harmful outcome in any situation and the extent of harm that results.

Risk management   control of hazards in any situation to minimise the possibility of a harmful outcome and limit its extent.

Seborrhoea   accumulation of skin, overactive sebaceous gland resulting in oily skin, scales or incrustation.

Speech and Language Therapist (SALT)   healthcare professional specialising in assessing and managing communication problems and swallowing difficulties.

Standard precautions   measures that reduce the risk of transmission of blood bourne pathogens.

Sterile field   area covered by a sterile sheet which serves as a clean space when performing an aseptic procedure.

Stridor   loud, harsh, high pitched respiratory sound usually heard on inspiration (due to partial obstruction) and common to young children.

Subcutaneous tissue   third layer of the skin containing fat, connective tissue, blood vessels, nerves and regulates temperature.

Sublingual   under the tongue.

Systolic pressure   contraction of the heart. Pressure exerted on the walls of the arteries representing the upper value of a blood pressure reading.

Tachycardia   rapid pulse rate.

Thermoregulatory centre   cells here are sensitive to blood flowing through the brain, and monitor and control body temperature.

Tympanic   meaning tympanum, thin semi-permeable membrane in the middle ear transmitting sound vibrations to the internal ear.

Vasoconstriction narrowing of the blood vessels.

Vasodilation widening of the blood vessels.

Violence an act where force is used to inflict personal harm.

Virus sub microscopic infectious agent unable to grow or reproduce outside a host.

Bibliography

Allen, K (2004) Principles and Limitations of Pulse Oximetry in Patient Monitoring, *Nursing Times* 100(4): 34 37.

APA Division 38 *What a Health Psychologist Does and How to Become One*, www.health-psych. org/articles/what_is.php

Argyle, J (1998) *The Psychology of Interpersonal Behaviour*, 5th edn. Penguin Press, Wandsworth.

Arinzon, Z, Feldman, J, Fidelman, JZ et al. (2004) Hypodermoclysis (Subcutaneous Infusion): Effective Mode of Treatment of Dehydration in Long Term Care Patients, *Archives of Gerontology and Geriatrics* 38(2): 167–173.

Arrowsmith, H (1993) Nursing Management of Patients Receiving a Nasogastric Feed, *British Journal of Nursing* 2(7): 1053–1058.

Ayliffe, GAJ et al. (2000) *Control of Hospital Infection: A Practical Handbook*, 4th edn. Arnold, London.

Baille, L (2001) *Developing Practical Nursing Skills*. Arnold, London.

Bandura, A (1986) *Social Foundations of Thought and Action: A Social Cognitive Theory*. Prentice Hall, Englewood Cliffs.

Banks, C (2005) Improving Your Communication Skills, *Nursing Times* 101(3): 48–49.

Barker, HM (2002) *Nutrition/Dietetics for Healthcare*, 10th edn. Churchill Livingstone, Edinburgh.

Baston, H (2001) Pulse and Respiratory Measurement, *The Practising Midwife* 4(11): 18–21.

Baston, H (2001) Blood Pressure Measurement, *The Practising Midwife* 9: 18–22.

Baston, H (2001) Temperature Measurement, *The Practising Midwife* 10: 19–22.

Bayer Diagnostics Europe (2004) *Your Practical Guide to Urine Analysis Bayer Healthcare*. Newbury, Berkshire.

Beauchamp, TL and Childress, JF (1992) *Principles of Biomedical Ethics*, 5th edn. Oxford University Press, Oxford.

Beck, SL (1996) *Mucositis*. In S Groemwuld et al. (eds) *Cancer Symptom Management*. Jones-Bartlett, Massachusetts.

Benjamin, M and Curtis, J (1992) *Ethics in Nursing*, 3rd edn. Oxford University Press, Oxford.

Bergstom, N et al. (1987) The Braden Scale for Predicting Pressure Sore Risk, *Nursing Research* 36(4): 205–210.

Beyea, SC and Nicholl, LH (1995) Administration of Medications via the Intramuscular Route: An Integrative Review of the Literature and Research Based Protocol for the Procedure, *Applied Nursing Research* 5(1): 23–33.

Blais, K and Bath, J (1992) Drug Calculation Errors of Bacculaureate Nursing Students, *Nurse Educator* 17(1): 12–15.

Blows, WT (2001) *The Biological Basis of Nursing: Clinical Observations*. Routledge, London.

Brammer, KW (1990) Management of Fungal Infections in Neutropenic Patients, *Haemtologyl Blood Transfusion* 33: 546–550.

Brooks, A (1994) Surgical Glove Perforation, *Nursing Times* 90(21): 60–62.

Brown, JM et al. (1997) *Challenges in Caring: Explorations in Nursing and Ethics.* Chapman and Hall, London.

Burkhardt, MA and Nathaniel, AK (2002) *Ethics and Issues in Contemporary Nursing,* 2nd edn. Delmar Thomson Learning, New York.

Burnham, W (1999) *Parenteral Nutrition.* In L Dougherty and J Lamn, (eds) *Intravenous Therapy in Nursing Practice.* Churchill Livingstone, Edinburgh.

Burnard, P and Chapman, C (2003) *Professional and Ethical Issues in Nursing,* 3rd edn. Balliere Tindall, Edinburgh.

Bursey, S et al. (2002) Hand Washing, *Professional Nurse* 16: 1417–1419.

Calliari, D (1995) The Relationship Between Calculation Test Given in Nursing Orientation and Medication Errors, *Journal of Continuing Education* 26(10): 11–14.

Caris-Verhallen, WMCM et al. (1999) Factors Related to Nurse Communication with Elderly People, *Journal of Advanced Nursing* 30(5): 1106–1117.

Charmorro, T (1990) Cancer of the Vulva and Vagina, *Semin Oncol Nurs* 6(3): 198–205.

Cohen, HA et al. (2002) Handwashing Patterns in Two Dermatology Clinics, *Dermatology* 205(4): 358–361.

Commission of the European Communities (2001) Council Directive on the Minimum Health and Safety Requirements for the Manual Handling of Loads Where There is a Risk of Back Injury to Workers 4th Directive 90/269/EEC, *Official Journal of the European Communities* 156: 9–13.

Copping, C (2005) Preventing and Reporting Drug Administration Errors, *Nursing Times* 101(33): 32–33.

Courts, S (1996) Monitoring Blood Pressure in Children, *Paediatric Nursing* 8(7): 25–27.

Crouch, D (2003) Easing the Pain of Constipation, *Nursing Times* 99(11): 23–25

Dairiki Shortliffe, LM (2002) *Urinary Tract Infections in Infants and Children.* In PC Walsh et al. (eds) *Campbell's Urology,* 8th edn. Saunders, Philadelphia.

Daeffler, R (1990) Oral Hygiene Measures for Patients with Cancer II, *Cancer Nurse* Dec 427–431.

Davidson, K and Barber, V (2004) Electronic Monitoring of Patients in General Wards, *Nursing Standard* 18(49): 42–46.

Davies, C (1989) Cleansing Rites and Wrongs, *Nursing Times* 95(43): 71–73.

Dealey, C (1989) *The Care of Wounds: A Guide for Nurses,* 2nd edn. Blackwell Science, Oxford.

DH (1997a) *Better Services for Vulnerable People* EC(97)62, C1(97)24.

DH (1997b) *The Coldicott Committee: Report on the Review of Patient-Identifiable Information.* DH, London.

DH (1998) *Partnership in Action: New Opportunities for Joint Working Between Health and Social Services – A Discussion Document.* DH, London.

DH (1999) *A National Service Framework for Mental Health.* DH, London.

DH (2000) *NHS Plan.* HMSO, London.

DH (2001a) *Withholding Treatment from Violent and Abusive Patients in NHS Trusts. NHS Zero Tolerance Zone HSC 2001/18.* Stationary Office, London.

DH (2001b) *12 Key Points on Consent: The Law in England.* HMSO, London.

DH (2003) *Confidentiality: NHS Code of Practice.* www.dh.gov.uk/publicationsandstatistics/publicationsandguidance

DH (2003) *PALS.* www.doh_gov.uk/PALS/downloads.htm

Dimitrovsky, L et al. (1998) Interpretation of Facial Expressions of Affect in Children with Learning Disability or Verbal or Non-Verbal Deficits, *Journal of Learning Disability* 31(3): 286–292; 312.

Dimond, B (2005) *Legal Aspects of Nursing*, 4th edn. Pearson, Harlow.

Dodd, MJ et al. (1996) Randomised Clinical Trial of Chlorhexidine Versus Placebo for Prevention of Oral Mucositis in Patients Receiving Chemotherapy, *Oncol Nurses Forum* 22(6): 921–927.

Donnelly, M (1999) The Benefits of Hypodermoclysis, *Nursing Standard* 13(52): 44–45.

Drever, J (1964) *A Dictionary of Psychology*. Penguin, Harmondsworth.

Eilers, J et al. (1988) Development, Testing and Application of the Oral Assessment Guide, *Oncology Nurse Forum* 15(3): 325–330.

Fairclough, N (1989) *Language and Power*. Longman, Harlow.

Feather, C (2001) Blood Pressure Measurement, *Nursing Times* 97(4): 33–34.

Ferguson, A (2005) Taking a Swab, *Nursing Times* 101(39): 26–27.

Ferguson, A (2005a) Administration of Oral Medication, *Nursing Times* 101(45): 24–25.

Ferguson-Clark, L and Williams, C (1998) Neurological Assessment in Children RCN Continuing Education Article 740, *Paediatric Nurse* 10(4): 29–35.

Flanagan, M (1998) The Characteristics and Formation of Granulation Tissue, *Journal of Wound Care* 7(10): 508–510.

Flores, A (2006) Appropriate Glove Use in the Prevention of Cross Infection, *Nursing Standard* 21(5): 45–48.

Flores, A and Pevalin, DJ (2006a) Healthcare Workers' Knowledge and Attitudes to Glove Use, *British Journal of Infection Control* 7(5): 18–22.

Flores, A and Pevalin, DJ (2006b) Healthcare Workers' Compliance with Glove Use and The Effect of Glove Use on Hand Hygiene Compliance, *British Journal of Infection Control* 7(6): 15–19.

Fredrickson, L (1999) Modes of Relaxing in a Caring Conversation: A Research Synthesis on Presence, Touch and Listening, *Journal of Advanced Nursing* 30(5): 1167–1176.

Garrard, C and Young, C (1998) Suboptimal Care of Patients Before Admission to Intensive Care, *British Medical Journal* 316(7148): 1841–1842.

Garwood-Gowers A, Tingle J and Wheat K (2005) *Contemporary Issues in Healthcare and Ethics*. Butterworth-Heinemann, Edinburgh.

Gatford, JD and Phillips, N (2006) *Nursing Calculations*, 7th edn. Churchill Livingstone, Edinburgh.

Getliffe, K and Dolman, M (eds) (2003) Incontinence in Perspective. In *Promoting Continence: A Clinical Research Resource*. Balliere Tindall, Edinburgh.

Gladstone, J (1995) Drug Administration Errors: A Study into the Factors Underlying the Occurrence and Reporting of Drug Errors in a District General Hospital, *Journal of Advanced Nursing* 22(4): 628–637.

Glasper, A and Richardson, J (eds) (2006) *A Textbook of Children's and Young People's Nursing*. Churchill Livingstone, London.

Gould, D (1994) Helping the Patient with Personal Hygiene, *Nursing Standard* 8(34): 30–22.

Gould, D (1994a) Making Sense of Hand Hygiene, *Nursing Times* 90(30): 63–64.

Gould, D, Smith, P, Payne, S and Aird, T (1999) Students' Expectations of Post Registration Degree Programme, *Journal of Advanced Nursing* 29: 1365–2648.

Gould, D (2002) Hand Decontamination, *Nursing Times* 98(46): 48–49.

Greenway, K and Hainsworth, T (2004) Is it Right to be Injecting the Dorsogluteal Site? *Nursing Times Practical Procedure Nursing Times* 100(47): 16.

Griffiths, J and Lewis, D (2002) Guidelines for Oral Care of Patients Who Are Dependent, Dysphagic or Critically Ill, *Journal of Disability and Oral Health* 3(1): 30–33.

Gross, RD (2001) *Psychology: The Science of Mind and Behaviour*, 4th edn. Hodder & Stoughton, London.

Hampton, S (2002) The Appropriate Use of Gloves to Reduce Allergies and Infection, *British Journal of Nursing* 11: 1120–1124.

Harris, AD et al. (2000) A Survey on Handwashing Practices and Opinions of Health Care Workers, *Journal of Hospital Infections* 45(4): 318–321.

Heath, H and McCormack, B (2002) *Nurses, the Body and Body Work.* In H Heath and I White (eds) *The Challenge of Sexualtiy in Health Care.* Blackwell, Oxford.

Health and Safety Executive (2000) *Simple Guide to the Lifting Operations and Lifting Equipment Regulations 1998.* HSE, Sudbury.

Heanue, M et al. (2003) *Manual Versus Powered Toothbrushing for Oral Health (Cochrane Review).* Cochrane Library Issue and Update Software, Oxford.

Henderson, V (1960) *Basic Principles of Nursing Care.* ICN, London.

Henderson, V (1966) *The Nature of Nursing: A Definition and its Implications for Practice, Research and Education.* Macmillan, New York.

HM Government (1998) *Data Protection Act.* TSO, London.

Higgins, D (2005) Nasogastric Tube Insertion, *Nursing Times* 101(37): 28–29.

Higgins, D (2005) Drug Calculations, *Nursing Times* 101(46): 24–25.

Hoban, V (2005) Wound Care What Every Nurse Should Know, *Nursing Times* 101(2): 20–22.

Holmes, S (1990) *Cancer Chemotherapy.* Lisa Sainsbury Foundation, Austin Cornish, London.

Holmes, S (2003) Undernutrition in Hospital Patients, *Nursing Standard* 17(19): 45–52.

Holmes, S and Mountain, E (1993) Assessment of Oral Status: Evaluation of Three Oral Assessment Guides, *Journal of Clinical Nursing* 2: 35–40.

Honey, P and Mumford, A (1992) *The Manual of Learning Styles,* 3rd edn. Peter Honey, Maidenhead.

Hood, LJ and Leddy, SK (2003) *Conceptual Bases of Professional Nursing,* 5th edn Lippincott, Philadelphia.

Hopkins, J (2004) Essentials of Newborn Skin Care, *British Journal of Midwifery* 12(5): 314–317.

Horton, R (1995) Handwashing: The Fundamental Infection Control Principle, *British Journal of Nursing* 4(16): 926–933.

International Council of Nurses (1987) *Position Statement.* ICNP, Geneva.

International Council of Nurses (1999) *International Classification for Nursing Practice Beta Version.* ICNP, Geneva.

International Council of Nurses (2002) *The ICN Definition of Nursing.* ICNP, Geneva.

Jeanes, A (2005) Infection Control: A Practical Guide to the Use of Hand Decontaminants, *Nursing Times* 100 (20): 46–48.

Jeanes, A (2005a) Putting on Gloves, *Nursing Times* 101(29): 28–29.

Jeanes, A (2005b) Using Alcohol Handrubs, *Nursing Times* 101(28): 28–29.

Jeanes, A (2005c) Handwashing, *Nursing Times* 101(27): 28–29.

Johns, C (2000) *Becoming a Reflective Practitioner.* Blackwell Science, London.

Johnson, R and Taylor, W (2005) *Skills for Midwifery Practice,* 2nd edn. Churchill Livingstone, Edinburgh.

Jones, A (1995) Reflective Process in Action: The Uncovering of the Ritual of Washing in Clinical Nursing Practice, *Journal of Clinical Nursing* 4(5): 283–288.

Kapborg, I (1994) Calculation and Administration of Drug Dosage by Swedish Nurses, Student Nurses and Physicians, *Journal for Quality in Health Care* 6(4): 389–395.

Kenworthy, N et al. (2001) *Common Foundation Studies in Nursing,* 3rd edn. Churchill Livingstone, Edinburgh.

King, S (1998) Decontamination of Equipment and the Environment, *Nursing Standard* 12(52): 57–63.

Kirby, C and Slevin, O (2003) Ethical Knowing: The Moral Ground of Nursing Practice. In L Basford and O Slevin (eds) *Theory and Practice of Nursing: An Integrated Approach to Caring Practice*, 2nd edn. Nelson Thorne, Cheltenham.

Kristhnasamy, M (1995) Oral Problems in Advanced Cancer, *European Journal of Cancer Care* 4: 173–177.

Lord, M (1997) Enteral Feeding Devices, *Nursing Clinics North America* 32(4): 685–704.

Lupton, D (1994) *Medicine as Culture: Illness, Disease and the Body in Western Societies*. Sage, London.

McGraw, A (2003) Nursing Patients with Gastrointestinal Disorders. In C Brooker and M Nicol (eds) *Nursing Adults. The Practice of Caring*. Mosby, Edinburgh.

McGuirk, V (2004) Skin Integrity Assessment in Neonates and Children, *Paediatric Nursing* 16(3): 15–19.

McHale, J and Tingle, J (2001) *Law and Nursing*, 2nd edn. Butterworth-Heinemann, Edinburgh.

McQuillan, P et al. (1998) Confidential Enquiry into Quality of Care Before Admission to Intensive Care, *British Medical Journal* 316(7148): 1853–1858.

McWhirter, JP and Pennington, CR (1994) Incidence and Recognition in Hospital, *British Medical Journal* 308: 945–948.

Maes, S and van Elderen, T (1998) Health Psychology and Stress. In M. Eysenck (ed.) *Psychology: An Integrated Approach*. Addison Wesley Longman, Harlow.

Mainstone, A (2005) Maintaining Infant Skin Health and Hygiene, *British Journal of Midwifery* 13(1): 44–47.

Mallik, M and McHale, J (1995) Support for Advocacy, *Nursing Times* 91(4): 28–30.

Mallick, M et al. (2004) *Nursing Knowledge and Practice Foundations for Decision Making*, 2nd edn. Balliere Tindall, Edinburgh.

Mansfield, S, Monaghan, H and Hall, J (1998) Subcutaneous Fluid Administration and Site Maintenance, *Nursing Standard* 13(12): 56, 59–62.

Marini, J and Wheeler, A (1997) *Critical Care Medicine: The Essentials*, 2nd edn. Williams and Wilkins, Baltimore.

Marr, PB et al. (1993) Bedside Terminal and Quality of Nursing Documentation, *Computers in Nursing* 11(4): 176–182.

Martin, EA (2002) *Concise Colour Medical Dictionary*. Oxford University Press, Oxford.

Mason, T and Whitehead, E (2003) *Thinking Nursing*. Oxford University Press, Maidenhead.

May, D (2000) Infection Control Must be the Priority for All, *British Journal of Nursing* 9(3): 254.

Miller, M and Dyson, M (1996) *Principles of Wound Care*. Macmillan, London.

Mooney, GP (2003a) Eye Care, *Nursing Times Handbook* 99(8): 7–8.

Mooney, GP (2003b) Mouth Care, *Nursing Times Handbook* 99(8): 13–14.

Mooney, GP (2003c) Temperature, *Nursing Times* 99(34): 2.

Mooney, GP (2003d) Pulse, *Nursing Times* 99(14): 29.

Mooney, GP Respiratory Assessment, *Nursing Times* 99(14): 29.

Mooney, GP Blood Pressure 2, *Nursing Times* 99(8): 7–8.

National Patient Safety Agency (2001) *Doing Less Harm*. DH, London.

NHS (2003) IT Q & A. www.nhs.uk/nhsmagazine/primarycare/it_qa.asp

NBPA/RCN (1998) *Guide to the Handling of Patients*, 4th edn. NBPA/RCN, London.

NHS Quality Improvement Scotland (2004) Working with Dependent Older People to Achieve Good Oral Care, *NHS/QIS* Scotland.

NHSE (1999) *Clinical Governance in London Region, Draft Template of Audit Risk Management Report for a Trust Board.* NHSE London Region, London.

Nicol, M et al. (2000) *Essential Nursing Skills.* Mosby, London.

NMC (2008) *The Code: Standards of Conduct, Performance and Ethics for Nurses.* NMC, London.

Norton, C (1996) The Causes and Management of Constipation, *British Journal of Nursing* 5(20): 1252–1258.

NMC (2004) *Standards of Proficiency for Pre-Registration Nursing Education.* NMC, London.

NPSA (2005) Patient Safety Information. www.npsa.nhs.uk/site/media/documents

Ogston-Tuck, S (2007) Legal Issues That Impact on Nursing Practice. In C Brooker and A Waugh (eds) *Foundations of Nursing Practice Fundamentals of Holistic Care.* Elsevier, Edinburgh.

Ottley, C (2002) Baby Tooth Care: A Forgotten Priority? *Nursing Standard* 16(18): 40–44.

Oxford English Dictionary (1989) *Oxford English Dictionary*, 2nd edn. Clarendon Press, Oxford.

Oxtoby, K (2005) Reaching a Clear Understanding, *Nursing Times* 101(20): 20–22.

Pergagallo-Dittko, V (1997) Rethinking Subcutaneous Injection Technique, *American Journal of Nursing* 97(5): 71–72.

Petit, D et al. (2000) Effectiveness of a Hospital Wide Programme to Improve Compliance with Hand Hygiene, *The Lancet* 356(9238): 1307–1312.

Pogson, D (2007) Genetic Knowledge Within an Ethical Framework. In R Hogston and BS Marjoram (eds) *Foundations of Nursing Practice: Leading the Way*, 3rd edn. Palgrave, Hampshire.

Pomfret, I (2000) Catheter Care in the Community, *Nursing Standard* 14(27): 46–51.

Porter, HJ (1994) Mouth Care in Cancer, *Nursing Times* 90(14): 27–29.

Pratt, RJ et al. (2001) Guidelines for Preventing Infections Associated with the Insertion and Maintenance of Short Term Indwelling Urethral Catheters in Acute Care, *Journal of Hospital Infection* 47(Suppl): S39–S46.

Raybould, LM (2001) Disposable Non Sterile Gloves: A Policy for Appropriate Usage, *British Journal of Nursing* 10(17): 1135–1141.

Rayner, D (2003) MRSA: An Infection Control Overview, *Nursing Standard* 17(45): 47–53.

Rennie-Meyer, K (2007) Preventing the Spread of Infection. In C Brooker and A Waugh (eds) *Foundations of Nursing Practice Fundamentals of Holistic Care.* Mosby, Philadelphia.

Riley, M (2000a) Establishing Nutritional Guidelines for Critically Ill Patients Part 1, *Professional Nurse* 17(10): 580–583.

Robinson, J (2001) Urethral Catheter Selection, *Nursing Standard* 15(25): 39–42.

Robinson, J (2004) A Practical Approach to Catheter Associated Problems, *Nursing Standard* 18(31): 38–42.

Rodger, MA and King, L (2000) Drawing up and Administering Intramuscular Injection: A Review of the Literature, *Journal of Advanced Nursing* 31(3): 574–582.

Roper, N. Logan, W and Tierney, AJ (1996) *The Elements of Nursing: A Nursing Model*, 3rd edn. Churchill Livingstone, Edinburgh.

Rosengren, K (2000) *Communication: An Introduction.* Sage, London.

Rowland, JH (1989) Developmental Stage and Adaptation: Child Adolescent Model. In JC Holland and JH Rowland (eds) *Handbook of Psycho-oncology.* Oxford University Press, New York.

RCN (2000) *Universal Precautions for the Control of Infection.* RCN, London.

RCN (2003) *Defining Nursing: Defining Nursing …* RCN, London.

Royal College of Paediatrics and Child Health (2002) *Position Statement on Injection Technique.* London.

Rush, M and Weatherall, A (2003) Temperature Measurement: Practice Guidelines, *Paediatric Nursing* 15(9): 25–28.

Sarafino, EP (2006) *Health Psychology: Biopsychosocial Interactions.* John Wiley and Sons Ltd, New Jersey.

Scottish Executive (2002) Preventing Infections Acquired While Receiving Healthcare 2002–2005. www. scotland.gov.uk/library5/health/preventinfect.pdf Available July 2006.

Secombe, I and Smith, G (1996) *In the Balance: RN Supply and Demand.* Institute for Employment Studies, Brighton.

Seedhouse, D (1988) *Ethics: The Heart of Health Care.* Wiley, Chichester.

Sharma, S et al. (2002) Guidelines: Are they Adhered to in Clinical Practice? *Journal of Clinical Governance* 10(2): 71–75.

Springhouse Corporation (1993) *Medication Administration and Intravenous Therapy Manual*, 2nd edn. Springhouse Corporation, Pennsylvania.

Springhouse Corporation (2000) *Nurse Practitioners Clinical Comparison.* Springhouse Corporation, Springhouse PA.

Sprunt, K et al. (1973) Antibacterial Effectiveness of Routine Handwashing. In J. Wilson (ed.) *Infection Control in Clinical Practice*, 2nd edn. Balliere Tindall, Edinburgh.

Steifel, K et al. (2000) Improving Oral Hygiene for the Seriously Ill Patient: Improving Research Based Practice, *MedSurg Nursing* 9: 40–43, 46.

Stevens-Haynes, J (2004) Pressure Ulcer Risk Assessment and Prevention, *British Journal of Community Nursing* 9(12): 540, 542–544.

Stevenson, T (2004) Achieving Best Practice in Routine Observation of Hospital Patients, *Nursing Times* 100(30): 34–36.

Sullivan, DH (1992) Risk Factors for Early Hospital Readmission in a Select Population of Geriatric Rehabilitation Patients: The Significance of Nutritional Status, *Journal of American Geriatrics Society* 40(8): 792–798.

Tait, D (2007) The Human Lifespan and Its Effect on Selecting Nursing Interventions. In C Brooker and A Waugh (eds) *Foundations of Nursing Practice Fundamentals of Holistic Care.* Mosby, Edinburgh.

Taylor, SE (1990) Health Psychology, *American Psychologist* 45(1): 40–50.

Taylor, J and Muller, D (1995) *Nursing Adolescents: Research and Psychological Perspectives.* Blackwell, Oxford.

Thomas, B (2001) *Manual of Dietetic Practice.* Blackwell Science, Oxford.

Thompson, IE (2006) *Nursing Ethics*, 5th edn. Churchill Livingstone, Edinburgh.

Tingle, J and Cribb, A (2003) *Nursing Law and Ethics*, 2nd edn. Blackwell, Oxford.

Trigg, E and Mohammed, TA (2006) *Practices in Children's Nursing. Guidelines for Hospital and Community*, 2nd edn. Churchill Livingstone, Edinburgh.

Trim, J (2004a) Clinical Skills: A Practical Guide to Working Out Drug Calculations, *British Journal of Nursing* 13(10): 602–606.

Trim, J (2004b) Performing a Comprehensive Physiological Assessment, *Nursing Times* 100(50): 38–42.

Trim, J (2005a) Respirations, *Nursing Times* 101(22): 30–31.

Trim, J (2005b) Monitoring Temperature, *Nursing Times* 101(20): 30–31.

Trim, J (2005c) Monitoring Pulse, *Nursing Times* 101(21): 30–31.

Trim, J (2005d) Blood Pressure, *Nursing Times* 101(02): 32–33.

UK Health Departments (1998) *Guidance for Clinical Healthcare Workers. Protection Against Infection with Bloodbourne Viruses, Recommendations of the Expert Advisory Group on AIDS and Advisory Group on Hepatitis.* DH, Wetherby.

Van Dongen, E (2001) It Isn't Something to Yodel About, but it Exists! Faeces, Nurses, Social Relations and Status Within a Mental Hospital, *Aging and Mental Health* 5(3): 205–215.

Waterlow, J (2005) *Pressure Ulcer Prevention Manual.* Waterlow, Taunton.

Watkins, S (2006) Improving Patient Nutrition Through Simple Initiatives, *Nursing Times* 102(1): 28–29.

Ward, S (2000) Evidence Based Practice and Infection Control, *British Journal of Nursing* 9(5): 267–271.

Williams, J (2005) Using an Alternative Device for Nasogastric Tubes, *Nursing Times* 101(35): 26–27.

Wilson, L (2005) Urinalysis, *Nursing Standard* 19(35): 51–54.

Windsor, JA et al. (1988) Wound Healing Response in Surgical Patients: Recent Food Intake is More Important than Nutritional Status, *British Journal of Surgery* 75:135–137.

WHO (1991) *Nursing in Action Project. Health for All Nursing Series No 2: Mission And Functions of the Nurse.* WHO, Copenhagen.

WHO (2003) *Practical Guidelines for Infection Control in Health Care Facilities.* WHO, Geneva. www.wpro. who.int/sars/doc/practicalguidelines/practical_guidelines.pdf

WHO (2006) Universal Precautions, Including Injections Safety. www.who.int/hiv/topics/precautions/ universalen/print

www.bapan.org.uk

www.bhf.org.uk/questions

www.bnf.org.uk

www.bpassoc.org.uk

www.continence-foundation.org.uk

www.diabetes.org.uk

www.digestive.niddk.nih.gov

www.edgehill.ac.uk/mtlr/presentations/OSCE-handwashing.html

www.eatwell.gov.uk

www.food.gov.uk

www.hpe.org.uk

www.icna.co.uk

www.nhscareers.nhs/details – Health Psychology Within the NHS

www.nice.org.uk

www.nice.org.uk/CG032quickrefguide

www.nursing-standard.co.uk

www.nutrition.org.uk

www.opsi.gov.uk/acts

www.phls.co.uk

www.rcn.org.uk

www.respiratory.co.uk

www.sustainweb.org

www.thinkfast.co.uk

www.vacine-administration.org.uk

Index

NOTE: Page numbers in *italic type* refer to procedure boxes.

ABPM (ambulatory blood pressure
    monitoring), 76
activist learners, 4
age
    and blood pressure, 74, 75
    and bowel movement, 129
    and faecal incontinence, 132
    and fluid intake, 113
    and heart rate, 71
    and hygiene needs, 90, 91, 93–4
    and respiratory rate/rhythm, 72, 73
    see also children
aggression, 17–20, *21–3*
alcohol-based hand rubs, 56–7, *60–1*
alopecia, 91
ambulatory blood pressure monitoring
    (ABPM), 76
anaesthetic gels, 126
aneroid blood pressure devices, 76
apical (apex) pulse, 71
aprons, 42
asepsis, 57
aseptic hand washing, 56
aseptic technique, 57–8, *61–2*, 129
    instances of use, 93, 110, 127, 166, 188
assessment
    of diarrhoea, 131
    nutritional, 106, 112
    of pressure ulcers, 184–6
    of risk, 12–13
auditory *see* ear
autonomic nervous system, 70
axillary temperature recordings, 68–9

back injury, 14
Bastable, S.B., 3–4
bladder, 123–4
bladder care, 125
    catheterisation, 125–9, *138–42*
    see also stoma care
blood pressure monitoring,
    74–6, *83–4*
blood spillages, *49*
bodily fluid spillages, *49–50*
body language, 27–8
bowel care, 129, 130–3, *142–4*
    see also stoma care

bowel movement
    constipation, 130, 133, *142 1*
    diarrhoea, 131, 133
    faecal incontinence, 131–2
    pathophysiology of, 129
Boyd, C., 181
Braden scale, 184, 185
bradycardia, 70, 79–80
British Hypertension Society, 75
Brown, D.L., 152
buccal drug administration, 157
burns, 15–16

cardiac output, 70
catheter bags, 128–9
catheter-associated urinary tract
    infections (CAUTIs), 126, 127, 128
catheters/catheterisation, 125–9, *138–42*
cerebral herniation, 79
children
    blood pressure, 74, 75
    drug administration, 156, 157, 158,
        159, 165
    faecal incontinence, 132
    heart rate, 71
    hygiene needs, 90, 91, 93–4
    neurological observations, 79
    respiratory rate/rhythm, 72, 73
choking, 17
clean technique, 58, 126
cleaning of wounds, 188
clinical practice, learning in, 8
clostridium difficile, 37, 57
colostomy, 134
colour coding of waste, 44, 45, 47
communication
    barriers to, 28–30
    conflict resolution, 19
    factors in, 27
    importance of, 26, 32–3
    non-verbal, 27–8
    record keeping, 30–2
    reflection exercises, 33–4
community, health and safety in, 19
community-acquired infections, 38
confidentiality, 31
conflict resolution, 19

consciousness, levels of, 77
consent, 155–6
constipation, 130, 133, *142 1*
continence, 124
continence care, 132–3
    see also bladder care; bowel care
controlled drugs (CDs), 150
core body temperature, 67
Cottrell, S., 6
covert drug administration, 155, 159
cultural beliefs, 89

dehydration, 114
deltoid injections, 170
dental care, 93–4
    see also oral hygiene
dentures, 99
dermis, 178
diarrhoea, 131, 133
diastolic blood pressure, 74
dorsogluteal injections, 171
dressings, 188–90
drinking
    factors affecting, 106–8
    see also hydrational needs; nutritional
        support
drug administration, 149, 155
    activities, 174–5
    errors in, 151–2
    injections, 159, 163–6, *175–6*
        activities, 167–73
    legislation and guidelines, 149–50
    professional responsibilities, 158–9
    routes of, 156–8, *159–61*
drug calculations, 152–5, 174–5
drugs
    and bowel movement, 130, 133
    controlled drugs, 150
    effects, 130
    storing, 150
Durkin, K., 5
duty of care, 11

ear
    drug administration via, 158
    temperature recording via, 68, *82*
ear care, 93

eating
  factors affecting, 106–8
  see also nutritional needs; nutritional
    support
elderly *see* older people
electrolyte imbalance, 107–8
elimination
  bowel care, 129
    constipation, 130, 133, *142–4*
    diarrhoea, 131
    faecal incontinence, 131–2
  bowel movement pathophysiology,
    129–30
  catheters, 125–9, *138–42*
  continence care, 132–3
  problems of, 124–5
  professional responsibilities, 137
  stoma care, 133–7, *145–6*
  urinary incontinence, 125
  urinary system functions, 123–5
encopresis, 132
enemas, 130, *142–3*
enteral feeding, 109, 110–12, *114–18*
epidermis, 178
essay writing, 6
Essential Skills Cluster document, 150
ethics
  of drug administration, 155–6
  and tube feeding, 112
exams, 6–7
experiential learning, 8
eye care, 92–3
eye protection, 43
eyes, pupil size and reaction, 78

hazard, 12
head lice, 91
Health Act (2006), 38
health and safety
  first aid, 15–17
  legislation, 13–14
  moving and handling, 14–15, *21*
  risk *see* risk assessment
  violence and aggression, 17–20, *21–3*
Health and Safety at Work Act (1974),
    13–14
Health and Safety at Work Regulations
    (1999), 14
heart rate, 70–1, *82*
Heins, T., 132
holistic approach, 89–90, 137
Honey, P., 4, 7
hospital-acquired infections, 36–7,
    39, 54–5
Hull, C., 4, 6
hydrational needs, 105, 112, 113–14, *119*
  factors affecting, 106–8
hydrophilic catheters, 127
hygiene needs, *99–101*
  ear and nose care, 93
  eye care, 92–3
  facial hair, 91–2, *102–3*
  hair care, 90–1
  holistic approach to, 89–90
  importance of, 88–9
  nail care, 92
  oral hygiene, 93–9, *101–2*
hypertension, 76, 79
hyperthermia, 69
  see also pyrexia
hypertonic infusions, 114
hyperventilation, 73
hypodermoclysis, 114
hypotension, 76
hypothermia, 69
hypotonic infusions, 114
hypoventilation, 73

IFIC (International Federation of
    Infection Control), 56
ileostomy, 134–5
incontinence, 124, 125, 131–2
infants *see* children
infection control, 37–9
  linen, 47–8
  protective equipment, 40–3
  sharps disposal, 46–7, 165
  spillages, 46, *48–50*
  standard precautions, 40
  waste management, 43–6
  see also aseptic technique; hand washing
Infection Control Nurses (ICNs), 38–9
infections, 36–7, 38, 180
  hospital acquired, 36–7, 39, 54–5
  UTIs, 126, 127, 128

information gathering, 5
inhaled medication, 158
injections, 159, 163–6, *175–6*
  activities, 167–73
interactive dressings, 188
intermittent catheterisation, 126–7
International Federation of Infection
    Control (IFIC), 56
interprofessional working, 137
intramuscular (I/M) injections, 164–5,
    170–3, *176*
isotonic infusions, 114

language, 28
laundry, 47–8
laxatives, 130
learning, 3–5, 8
  see also study skills
lectures, 5
legislation/guidelines
  drug administration, 149–50
  health and safety, 13–14
  infection control, 38
  waste management, 44
lifting *see* moving and handling
Lifting Operations and Lifting
    Equipment Regulations (LOLER)
    (1998), 14
limb power, 78–9
linen, 47–8
local drug administration routes, 156

Main, A., 5
male catheterisation, 126, 127–8
malnutrition, 106
masks, 42–3
medical record keeping, 30–2
medication *see* drug administration; drugs
Mental Health Act (1983), 156
Mental Health Bill (2006), 156
mercury sphygmanometers, 76
mercury spillages, *50*
methicillin resistant staphylococcus
    aureus (MRSA), 36–7, 57
motor functioning, 78–9
mouth care *see* oral hygiene
moving and handling, 14–15, *21*
Moving and Handling Operations
    Regulations (1992), 14
MRSA (methicillin resistant
    staphylococcus aureus), 36–7, 57
Mumford, A., 4, 7
muscle bunch technique, 164

nail care, 92
naso-gastric (NG) tubes, 109,
    110–11, *114–17*
needle stick injuries, 165
needles, 163, 164, 165
  sharps disposal, 46–7, 165

Garnham, P., 18
Glasgow Coma Score (GCS), 77, 79
gloves, 41–2, 55, *62–3*
Gohel, S., 181
gowns, 42

hair care, 90–1
  and drying, 55
hand washing, 37, 42, 54–7, *59–60*
handling and moving, 14–15, *21*
hats, 43

neurolinguistic programme (NLP)
    models, 27
neurological observations, 76–7, 80, *85*
    levels of consciousness, 77
    motor and sensory function, 78–9
    pupil size and reaction, 78
    scenarios, 80–1
NHS Modernisation Agency, 133
NMC (Nursing and Midwifery
    Council), 11–12
non-touch technique *see* aseptic
    technique; clean technique
non-verbal communication, 27–8
nose care, 93
nosocomial (hospital acquired)
    infections, 36–7, 39, 54–5
note taking, 5
NPSA (National Patient Safety Agency),
    13, 151, 152
nutritional assessment and screening,
    106, 112
nutritional needs, 105
    factors affecting eating and drinking,
        106–8
    and professional responsibility, 112
    see also hydrational needs
nutritional support, 108–14
    feeding, 109–12, *114–18*, 120

observations *see* neurological
    observations; vital signs
older people, 113, 132
oral drug administration, 157, *159–61*
oral hydration, 113
oral hygiene, 93–9, *101–2*
oral temperature recordings, 68, 69
oxygen saturations, 73–4, *84*

parenteral feeding, 111
passive dressings, 188
percutaneous endoscopic gastrostomy
    (PEG) tube, 109, 111, *117–19*
perianal area, 90
personal protective equipment, 40–3,
    55, *62–3*
pharmacodynamics, 152
pharmacokinetics, 152
poisons, 16–17
pragmatist learners, 4
presentations, 6
pressure ulcers, 183–7, *192*
professional responsibilities
    and drug administration, 158–9
    and elimination needs, 137
    and nutritional needs, 112
    violence, aggression and, 18–20
    and wound management, 190
protective equipment, 40–3, 55, *62–3*

Provision and Use of Work Equipment
    Regulations (PUWER) (1998), 14
pulse oximetry, 73–4, *84*
pulse recording, 70–1, *82*
pupil size and reaction, 78
pyrexia, 69, 80

record keeping, 30–2
rectal drug administration, *144*, 157–8
rectal temperature recordings, 68, 69
rectus femoris injections, 173
reflection, 8–9
reflector learners, 4
regulations *see* legislation/guidelines
report writing, 7
Reporting of Incidents, Diseases and
    Dangerous Occurences Regulations,
    (RIDDOR) (1995), 14
respiratory rate recording, 71–3, *83*
reticular-activating system (RAS), 78
risk assessment, 12–13, 14, 19, 41
    of diarrhoea, 131
    and nutrition, 106, 112
    of pressure ulcers, 184–6
risk management, 11–12, 13, 19–20
Ritchie, K., 132
rule of nines, 16

scalds, 15–16
self-catheterisation, 126–7
sensory functioning, 78–9
sharps disposal, 46–7, 165
shaving, 91, *102–3*
skin
    cleaning prior to injection, 165
    features and functions of, 178–9
    pressure ulcers, 183–7, *192*
    wound healing, 180–2
    wound management, 188–90, *190–2*
skin barriers, 136–7
skin care basics, 179
skin pinch approach, 164
social beliefs, 89
social hand washing, 56
solutions, in stoma care, 136–7
sphygmanometers, 76
spillages, 46, *48–50*
standard precautions, 40
    linen, 47–8
    protective equipment, 40–3
    sharps disposal, 46–7, 165
    spillages, 46, *48–50*
    waste management, 43–6
sterile *see* aseptic technique
stoma bags, 135
stoma care, 133–7, *145–6*
stridor, 73
stroke volume, 70

study skills, 3, 5–9
subcutaneous (S/C) infusions, 114, *119*
subcutaneous (S/C) injections, 164, *175*
subcutaneous tissue, 178
sublingual drug administration, 157
suppositories, 130, *144*, 157
suprapubic catheters, 127
surface body temperature, 67
syringes, 163
systemic drug administration routes, 156
systolic blood pressure, 74

tachycardia, 70
temperature recording, 67–70, *82*
theorist learners, 4
Thomas-Hess, C., 179
topical medications, 158
tube feeding *see* enteral feeding;
    parenteral feeding
tympanic temperature recordings, 68, *82*

universal precautions *see* standard
    precautions
urinary incontinence, 125
    see also catheters/catheterisation
urinary system, functions of, 123–5
urinary tract infections (UTIs), 126,
    127, 128
urostomy, 135

vasoconstriction, 68
vasodilation, 68
vastus lateralis injections, 173
ventrogluteal injections, 172
violence and aggression, 17–20, *21–3*
vital signs, 67, 80
    blood pressure monitoring, 74–6, *83–4*
    measuring and recording, 79–80
    oxygen saturations, 73–4, *84*
    pulse recording, 70–1, *82*
    respiratory rate recording, 71–3, *83*
    scenarios, 80–1
    temperature recording, 67–70, *82*

waste management and disposal, 43–6
Waterlow scale, 184, 186
wound management, *190–2*
    cleaning, 188
    dressings, 188–90
    pressure ulcers, 184–7
    professional responsibilities, 190
wounds, 179
    healing process, 180–2
    pressure ulcers, 183–7, *192*
writing essays, 6
writing reports, 7

Z track approach, 164